Exploring the Science Behind Intermittent Fasting.

How Understanding Your Body's Metabolic Processes Can Revolutionise Weight Management"

Jason Stephens

TABLE OF CONTENTS

Introduction to Intermittent Fasting.

Certainly! Here is a prologue to discontinuous fasting: Irregular fasting (IF) is a dietary method that includes exchanging times of eating and fasting. Dissimilar to conventional weight control plans that emphasise on what food varieties to eat or stay away from, irregular fasting focuses on when you eat. It's anything but another idea; people have worked on fasting for a really long time considering multiple factors, including strict observances and social practices. At its center, discontinuous fasting works on the rule of cycling between times of eating and fasting, determined to streamline metabolic cycles and advancing different medical advantages. During the fasting time frames, the body goes through physiological changes that can prompt enhancements in weight the board, metabolic wellbeing, and prosperity. There are a few distinct techniques for irregular fasting, each with its own interesting way to deal with timing eating windows and fasting periods. These strategies incorporate time-limited eating, substitute day fasting, intermittent fasting, and that's only the tip of the iceberg. The adaptability of discontinuous fasting permits people to pick a technique that best suits their way of life and objectives. As of late, discontinuous fasting has gained prominence because of its capability to support weight reduction, further develop metabolic markers, for example, glucose and insulin levels, and even improve mental capability. It's fundamental for approaching discontinuous fasting with wariness and designed it to individual necessities, considering variables like clinical history, way of life, and healthful prerequisites. Irregular fasting offers a clever way to deal with sustenance and wellbeing that goes past just counting calories or limiting specific nutrition classes. By understanding the standards behind discontinuous fasting and what it means for the body's metabolic cycles, people can outfit its capability to alter their way of dealing with weight on the board and wellbeing.

- Characterizing Discontinuous Fasting.

Characterising discontinuous fasting (IF) includes figuring it out as a dietary example that shifts back and forth between times of eating and fasting. Not at all, like conventional calorie limitation abstains from food, irregular fasting centres on when to eat instead of what to eat. There are different irregular fasting techniques. However, they regularly include cycling between times of fasting and eating. Normal methodologies include:

1. Time-Confined Eating (TRE): This technique includes limiting eating to a particular window of time every day, like an 8-hour term, with the leftover hours assigned for fasting.

2. Substitute Day Fasting (ADF): With ADF, people shift back and forth between

long stretches of customary eating and fasting days, where either no food is devoured or an essentially diminished calorie admission is noticed.

3. Intermittent Fasting: This approach includes longer fasting periods, regularly enduring a few days or even as long as seven days, scattered with times of typical eating. Discontinuous fasting doesn't endorse explicit food sources to eat or keep away from, yet rather centers on when to eat them. During fasting periods, people avoid polishing off calories, however non-caloric refreshments like water, tea, and espresso are typically allowed. The essential aim of irregular fasting is to take advantage of the body's metabolic instruments, advancing fat consuming and other physiological cycles that can prompt different medical advantages, including weight reduction, further developed insulin responsiveness, decreased irritation, and upgraded cell fix. It's critical to note that irregular fasting may not be appropriate for everybody, and

individual factors, for example, ailments, drug use, and way of life, ought to be viewed as prior to beginning any fasting routine. Talking with a medical care proficient or enrolled dietitian can help decide whether discontinuous fasting is fitting and safe for a singular's particular conditions.

- Verifiable Foundation and Social Practices.

The authentic foundation and social works on encompassing irregular fasting give important experiences into its beginnings and a far-reaching reception across various social orders over the entire course of time.

1. Old Roots: Fasting has been rehearsed for quite a long time, with establishes in old societies and strict customs. Many civic establishments, including old Greeks, Romans, and Egyptians, integrated fasting into their otherworldly practices for decontamination, retribution, and profound edification.

2. Strict Observances: Different religions integrate fasting into their customs and observances. For instance, fasting during Ramadan is a basic piece of Islamic practice,

where Muslims swear off food and drink from first light until nightfall all month long. Fasting is seen during the Loaned in Christianity and Yom Kippur in Judaism, among other strict events.

3. Clinical Customs: Fasting has likewise been used in conventional clinical frameworks, like Ayurveda and Customary Chinese Medication (TCM), for helpful purposes. Old healers perceived the body's capacity to recuperate itself during times of fasting and endorsed fasting as a treatment for different sicknesses.

4. Investigation and Logical Request: The advantages of fasting drawn in logical premium in the mid twentieth 100 years, with analysts investigating its impacts on wellbeing and life span. Trailblazers in the field, like Dr. Otto Buchinger and Dr. Walter Longo, led examinations on fasting and its expected restorative applications.

5. Current Resurgence: In late many years, discontinuous fasting has encountered a resurgence in fame, filled by logical examination featuring its potential medical advantages. Books, articles, and online assets have added to the boundless reception of irregular fasting as a weight the board procedure and direction for living. Understanding the verifiable setting and social meaning of discontinuous fasting can give a more profound appreciation to its job in human culture and it's getting through request as a dietary practice. Besides, perceiving the assorted social customs and profound convictions related to fasting highlights its widespread importance across various civic establishments and time spans.

Chapter One
The Science of Fasting.

The science of fasting digs into the multifaceted metabolic cycles that happen inside the body when food admission is limited. Understanding these instruments reveals insight into what fasting can mean for different parts of wellbeing and prosperity.

1. Digestion and Energy Equilibrium: When food is eaten, separated into supplements give energy to cell capabilities. During fasting, the body shifts from utilizing glucose got from food to using put away energy sources, like glycogen and fat, to meet its energy needs. Chemicals managed this metabolic switch, like insulin, glucagon, and adrenaline.

2. Hormonal Reactions to Fasting: Fasting triggers an outpouring of hormonal changes that assist with preparing put away energy and keep up with glucose levels. Insulin levels decline, permitting put away glycogen to be separated into glucose, while glucagon and adrenaline increment, invigorating glucose from the liver and advancing fat breakdown for energy.

3. Autophagy and Cell Fix: Fasting invigorates autophagy, a cell interaction that includes the breakdown and reusing of harmed or useless cell parts. This interaction helps eliminate poisons and advance cell fix and recovery, which might have suggestions for maturing, sickness anticipation, and life span.

4. Ketosis and Ketogenesis: Expanded times of fasting or starch limitation can prompt the development of ketone bodies through an interaction called ketogenesis. Ketones act as an elective fuel hotspot for the cerebrum and different tissues when glucose

accessibility is restricted. This metabolic state, known as ketosis, is related to different medical advantages, including upgraded mental capability and worked on metabolic wellbeing.

5. Fiery and Oxidative Pressure Decrease: Fasting has been displayed to lessen markers of aggravation and oxidative pressure, which are embroiled in the advancement of ongoing illnesses like heftiness, type 2 diabetes, and cardiovascular sickness. By advancing cell fix and diminishing provocative cycles, fasting might assist with moderating sickness risk and advance wellbeing. The science of fasting features the body's surprising skill to adjust to changes in supplement accessibility and use put away energy stores to keep up with metabolic homeostasis. By understanding these hidden instruments, scientists can clarify the physiological impacts of fasting and investigate its possible restorative applications for wellbeing advancement and infection counteraction.

- Grasping Digestion.

Understanding digestion is vital for appreciating how our bodies cycle and use energy from the food varieties we devour. Here is an outline:

1. Nuts and bolts of Digestion: Digestion alludes to the mind-boggling set of substance responses that happen in the body to keep up with life. It includes two principal processes: catabolism, where atoms are separated to deliver energy, and anabolism, where particles are combined to assemble new cell parts.

2. Energy Equilibrium: Digestion assumes a focal part in energy balance, which is the harmony between the energy devoured through food and refreshments and the energy used through basal metabolic rate (BMR), actual work, and other metabolic cycles. At the point when energy admission surpasses use, the overabundance is put away as fat; when energy admission is

deficient, put away fat is utilized to satisfy energy needs.

3. Macronutrient Digestion: The three essential macronutrients carbs, fats, and proteins are processed distinctively to give energy: - Sugars are separated into glucose, which can be utilized quickly for energy or put away as glycogen in the liver and muscles.

- Fats are separated into unsaturated fats and glycerol, which are used for energy creation or put away in fat tissue.

- Proteins are separated into amino acids, which can be utilized for energy or for building and fixing tissues.

4. Job of Chemicals: Chemicals assume a key part in managing digestion by flagging the body to one or the other increment or lessening energy use and capacity. For instance, insulin advances the take-up of glucose by cells and works with its capacity

as glycogen or fat, while glucagon invigorates the breakdown of glycogen into glucose to raise glucose levels.

5. Factors Affecting Digestion: Metabolic rate the rate at which the body uses energy can be impacted by different elements, including hereditary qualities, age, orientation, body arrangement, and action level. Bulk, for instance, increments metabolic rate since muscle tissue requires more energy to keep up with than fat tissue.

6. Suggestions for Weight The executives: Understanding digestion is fundamental for successful weight the board techniques. By enhancing metabolic wellbeing through adjusted sustenance, customary actual work, and way of life changes, people can uphold their body's capacity to keep a sound weight and, in general, prosperity. In outline, digestion is a unique cycle that directs energy balance and is impacted by different elements. By understanding the basics of digestion, people can pursue informed

decisions to help their wellbeing and wellness objectives.

- Hormonal Reactions to Fasting.

Hormonal reactions to fasting assume an urgent part in controlling energy digestion and keeping up with glucose levels during times of food hardship. Here outlines the key hormonal changes that happen:

1. Insulin: the pancreas delivers insulin because of rising blood glucose levels after a dinner. Its essential capability is to work with the take-up of glucose into cells for energy creation or capacity as glycogen in the liver and muscles. During fasting, insulin levels decline, permitting put away glycogen to be separated into glucose to keep up with glucose levels.

2. Glucagon: Glucagon, additionally delivered by the pancreas, has the contrary impact of insulin. It animates the breakdown of glycogen put away in the liver into glucose, which is delivered into the

circulation system to raise glucose levels. Glucagon levels increment during fasting to guarantee a consistent inventory of glucose for fundamental physical processes.

3. Adrenaline (Epinephrine): The adrenal organs deliver adrenaline considering pressure or low glucose levels. During fasting, adrenaline levels ascend to invigorate the breakdown of glycogen into glucose and advance unsaturated fats from fat tissue for energy creation. Adrenaline additionally helps increment readiness and energy consumption to help endurance during times of food shortage.

4. The pituitary organ emits Development Chemical: Development chemical (GH)and assumes a part in advancing development, digestion, and tissue fix. During fasting, GH levels increment to assist with protecting slender bulk and invigorate fat breakdown for energy. GH likewise improves the body's capacity to involve unsaturated fats as fuel,

saving glucose for tissues that depend on it, like the mind.

5. Cortisol: Cortisol, frequently alluded to as the pressure chemical, is delivered by the adrenal organs considering different stressors, including fasting. Cortisol activates energy holds by advancing the breakdown of protein and fat stores for fuel. While cortisol levels normally ascend during fasting, delayed rise can inconveniently affect digestion and wellbeing. These hormonal reactions to fasting are finely organized to guarantee a consistent stock of energy for crucial organs and tissues, while likewise protecting fit bulk and metabolic capability. Understanding how these chemicals cooperate during fasting can give bits of knowledge into the body's versatile reactions to times of food shortage and may illuminate methodologies for upgrading metabolic wellbeing and weight of the executives.

Chapter Two
Autophagy and Cell Fix, Kinds of Discontinuous Fasting.

Autophagy, a phone cycle urgent for keeping up with cell wellbeing and capability, is progressively perceived for its part in advancing life span and prosperity, particularly during fasting. Here outlines autophagy and its importance for cell fix:

1. What is Autophagy? Autophagy, got from the Greek words "auto" (self) and "phagy" (eating), is a profoundly monitored cell process liable for the corruption and reusing of harmed or useless cell parts. It includes the arrangement of particular designs called autophagosome, which immerse and sequester cell material for debasement by lysosomes.

2. Key Parts of Autophagy: The course of autophagy includes a few key parts, including:

- Commencement: Autophagy is started considering different cell stressors, like supplement hardship, oxidative pressure, or protein totals.

- Arrangement of Autophagosomes: Twofold film vesicles called autophagosome structure around cell material focused on for corruption.

- Combination with Lysosomes: Autophagosomes meld with lysosomes, acidic organelles containing hydrolytic catalysts, to shape autolysosomes, where the overwhelmed material is corrupted.

- Reusing: Debasement items, like amino acids, unsaturated fats, and sugars, are reused and used to help cell digestion and energy creation.

3. Job of Autophagy in Cell Fix: Autophagy assumes a pivotal part in keeping up with cell homeostasis by eliminating harmed organelles, misfolded proteins, and poisonous totals that gather during typical cell digestion or because of stress. By getting out these cells "garbage" parts,

autophagy forestalls the collection of destructive substances and advances cell wellbeing and life span.

4. Effect of Fasting on Autophagy: Fasting is a strong inducer of autophagy, essentially because of supplement hardship and energy limitation. During fasting, the body's energy saves are drained, setting off autophagy for of reusing cell parts to produce energy and backing metabolic cycles. Studies have showed how fasting can upgrade autophagic movement in different tissues, including the liver, cerebrum, and muscles, which might add to its wellbeing advancing impacts.

5. Medical advantages of Autophagy Activation: Actuation of autophagy has been connected to various medical advantages, including:
- Worked on cell capability and life span -
Insurance against age-related illnesses, like neurodegenerative problems, disease, and metabolic disorder

- Upgraded pressure obstruction and transformation to natural difficulties
- Advancement of tissue fix and recovery In synopsis, autophagy is a key cell process engaged with keeping up with cell homeostasis and advancing cell fix and reestablishment.

Understanding the job of autophagy and its enactment during fasting gives bits of knowledge of the instruments basic the medical advantages related to irregular fasting and may illuminate systems for advancing life span and prosperity.
- Time-Confined Eating. Irregular fasting envelops a few distinct methodologies, each changing in the length and recurrence of fasting periods. Here are the absolute most normal kinds of irregular fasting:
1. Time-Confined Eating (TRE): This technique includes restricting the everyday eating window to a particular time span, ordinarily going from 8 to 12 hours, with the excess hours assigned for fasting. For instance, a well-known approach is the 16/8

strategy, where people quick for 16 hours and eat inside an 8-hour window every day.

2. Substitute Day Fasting (ADF): With ADF, people switch back and forth between fasting days and non-fasting days. On fasting days, calorie admission is seriously confined (e.g., to 500-600 calories) or totally kept away from, while on non-fasting days, people eat not indispensable.

3. 5:2 Eating regimen: In this method, people eat typically for five days of the week and confine calorie admission to around 500-600 calories on two non-sequential days. These fasting days are regularly dispersed separated during the week.

4. Intermittent Fasting: Occasional fasting includes longer fasting periods, going from 24 hours to a few days or even as long as seven days, blended with times of typical eating. Models incorporate the 24-hour quick, where people cease from eating for an entire day, and multi-day diets, for example, the 3-day water quick or the 5-day fasting imitating diet.

5. Eat-Stop-Eat: This strategy includes fasting for an entire 24-hour time span more than once per week, regularly from supper one day to supper the following day. Water, natural tea, and other non-caloric refreshments are permitted during the fasting time frame.

6. Hero Diet: Propelled by old champion societies, this approach includes fasting for most the day and consuming one huge feast, normally at night, during a 4-hour eating window. The fasting time frame goes on for close to 20 hours, during which modest quantities of crude foods grown from the ground or protein-rich bites might be eaten.

7. Unconstrained Feast Skipping: A few people practice irregular fasting by suddenly skipping dinners when they are not eager or when it is helpful. This adaptable method considers changeability in the fasting term and recurrence in view of individual inclinations and way of life. Each kind of irregular fasting has its remarkable attributes and may interest various people considering their objectives, inclinations, and way of life

factors. Exploring different avenues regarding various methodologies can assist people with tracking down a fasting routine that meets their requirements and advances adherence over the long haul. It's fundamental to pick a discontinuous fasting strategy that is reasonable and viable with wellbeing and prosperity.

- Substitute Day Fasting.

Substitute Day Fasting (ADF) is a discontinuous fasting approach that includes shifting back and forth between fasting days and non-fasting days. This is the secret:

1. Fasting Days: On fasting days, people consume either no calories or an essentially diminished calorie consumption, frequently around 500-600 calories. A few varieties of ADF consider one little dinner or nibble during fasting days, while others advocate for complete fasting. Water, natural tea, and other non-caloric refreshments are permitted to assist with controlling craving and remain hydrated.

2. Non-Fasting Days: On non-fasting days, people eat not obligatorily, meaning they can eat as they typically would with next to no particular limitations on food decisions or calorie admission. Non-fasting days give an amazing chance to appreciate normal dinners and fulfill hunger without the imperatives of fasting.

3. Recurrence: The recurrence of fasting and non-fasting days can change contingent upon individual inclinations and objectives. Certain individuals decide to follow a severe ADF routine with substituting fasting and non-fasting days over time, while others might select a changed form with less fasting days or discontinuous fasting on specific days of the week.

4. Benefits: Substitute Day Fasting has been related to different medical advantages, including weight reduction, worked on metabolic wellbeing, and decreased irritation. By shifting back and forth between times of fasting and customary eating, ADF can make a calorie shortfall, prompting weight reduction after some time. Also, ADF might further develop insulin responsiveness, lipid profiles, and markers of cardiovascular wellbeing.

5. Challenges: While ADF can be compelling for weight reduction and working on metabolic wellbeing, it may not be appropriate for everybody. Certain individuals might find it trying to stick to

severe fasting days, particularly during the underlying change time frame. Fasting for stretched out periods might prompt sensations of appetite, exhaustion, and peevishness, which can influence everyday exercises and prosperity.

6. Contemplations: It's crucial to approach ADF with alert and think about individual factors like clinical history, dietary necessities, and way of life inclinations. Talking with a medical services proficient or enrolled dietitian can help decide whether ADF is proper and ok for a singular's particular conditions. Substitute Day Fasting offers an organized way to deal with irregular fasting that can be powerful for weight reduction and further developing metabolic wellbeing when followed reliably and joined with a fair eating regimen and normal active work.

- Intermittent Fasting.

Occasional fasting, otherwise called delayed fasting or expanded fasting, includes longer fasting periods that reach out past the normal everyday discontinuous fasting regimens. Here outlines occasional fasting:

1. Term: Occasional fasting commonly includes fasting for broadened periods, going from 24 hours to a few days or even as long as seven days. In contrast to irregular fasting, where fasting periods are more limited and sprinkled with eating windows, occasional fasting stretches out the fasting span to advance further metabolic and cell transformations.

2. Water Fasting: One normal way to deal with intermittent fasting is water fasting, where people polish off just water and non-caloric drinks during the fasting time frame. Water fasting considers total abstention

from food while guaranteeing satisfactory hydration and electrolyte balance.

3. Fasting Imitating Diet (FMD): One more variety of intermittent fasting is the fasting mirroring diet, which includes consuming an extremely low-calorie and supplement thick eating regimen for a predetermined number of days.

The FMD means to emulate the physiological impacts of fasting while giving fundamental supplements to help metabolic cycles and limit the distress related to complete fasting.

4. Benefits: Occasional fasting has been related to different medical advantages, including weight reduction, worked on metabolic wellbeing, upgraded cell fix and recovery, and life span. By advancing further ketosis and autophagy, occasional fasting might offer extra metabolic and cell benefits contrasted with more limited, discontinuous fasting regimens.

5. Contemplations: While intermittent fasting can be successful in advancing weight reduction and working on metabolic

wellbeing, it may not be appropriate for everybody. Drawn out fasting can prompt supplement lacks, electrolyte uneven characters, and possible unfavorable impacts, particularly in people with basic ailments or the individuals who are pregnant, breastfeeding, or underweight. It's crucial to approach occasional fasting with alert and under the direction of a medical services proficient or enrolled dietitian, especially for longer fasting lengths.

6. Security and Checking: During intermittent fasting, it's pivotal to screen hydration status, electrolyte equilibrium, and prosperity. Satisfactory hydration and supplementation with electrolytes, like sodium, potassium, and magnesium, might be important in forestall drying out and keep up with physiological capability. Occasional fasting offers a more escalated way to deal with fasting that might give extra metabolic and cell benefits contrasted with discontinuous fasting. It requires cautious thought and observing to guarantee security

and adequacy, particularly for delayed fasting lengths.

Chapter Three
Advantages of Irregular Fasting.

Irregular fasting (IF) has gained fame as of late because of its potential medical advantages. Here are a portion of the key advantages related to discontinuous fasting:

1. Weight reduction and Fat Loss: Intermittent fasting can advance weight reduction by making a calorie shortage through decreased calorie consumption during fasting periods. Irregular fasting might upgrade fat consuming and protect fit bulk, prompting more noteworthy fat misfortune contrasted with consistent calorie limitation.

2. Worked on Metabolic Wellbeing: Discontinuous fasting has been displayed to work on different markers of metabolic wellbeing, including insulin responsiveness, glucose control, and lipid profiles. By controlling insulin levels and advancing glucose and lipid digestion, irregular fasting might diminish the gamble of type 2

diabetes, metabolic disorder, and cardiovascular illness.

3. Improved Autophagy and Cell Repair: Fasting triggers autophagy, a cell cycle that advances the evacuation of harmed or useless cell parts and invigorates cell fix and recovery. Upgraded autophagy may add to life span, worked on resistant capability, and insurance against age-related infections.

4. Diminished Aggravation: Irregular fasting makes mitigating impacts, as proven by decreases in provocative markers like C-receptive protein (CRP) and interleukin-6 (IL-6). By decreasing constant aggravation, irregular fasting might bring down the gamble of provocative illnesses and work on wellbeing.

5. Mental Advantages: A few examinations recommend that discontinuous fasting might improve mental capability, memory, and cerebrum wellbeing. Fasting-actuated ketosis, expanded creation of cerebrum inferred neurotrophic factor (BDNF), and improved mitochondrial capability are

remembered to add to these mental advantages.

6. Life span: Irregular fasting has been related to expanded life expectancy and life span in creature studies. While more examination is expected to decide its consequences for human life expectancy, discontinuous' ability too fast to work on metabolic wellbeing, lessen oxidative pressure, and advance cell fix and recovery might add to life span and sound maturing.

7. Effortlessness and Accommodation: Irregular fasting is easy to carry out and doesn't need severe calorie counting or muddled feast plans. It offers adaptability in food decisions and feast timing, making it helpful for some individuals to integrate into their way of life. It's vital to note that singular reactions to discontinuous fasting might change, and not all people might encounter similar advantages. Irregular fasting may not be appropriate for everybody, particularly those with specific ailments or dietary limitations. Talking with a medical care proficient or enrolled

dietitian is prescribed prior to beginning any fasting routine to guarantee security and viability.

- Weight reduction and Body Creation Changes.

Discontinuous fasting (IF) has been broadly read up for its adequacy in advancing weight reduction and great changes in body synthesis. This is the way discontinuous fasting can add to weight reduction and body synthesis changes:

1. Calorie Limitation: Discontinuous fasting commonly brings about a decrease in calorie consumption, by shortening the eating window or fasting for broadened periods. This calorie limitation makes a negative energy balance, prompting weight reduction over the long run.

2. Improved Fat Consuming: During fasting periods, the body's insulin levels decline, permitting put away fat to be activated and used for energy. Irregular fasting advances lipolysis, the breakdown of fat stores, and increments unsaturated fat oxidation, prompting more prominent fat consuming and a decrease in muscle to fat ratio.

3. Conservation of Fit Bulk: Not at all like consistent calorie limitation slims down, which can prompt muscle misfortune alongside fat misfortune, discontinuous fasting has been displayed to save slender bulk. Studies propose that irregular fasting might upgrade muscle protein union and advance the maintenance of bulk, bringing about a better body synthesis with a higher extent of lean tissue to fat tissue.

4. Metabolic Transformations: Irregular fasting can prompt metabolic variations that help reduce weight reduction and body structure changes. These variations remember upgrades for insulin responsiveness, glucose control, and chemical guideline, which add to improved fat digestion and metabolic adaptability.

5. Diminished Gut Fat: Irregular fasting has been displayed to explicitly target instinctive fat, the fat put away around the stomach organs, which is related to an expanded gamble of metabolic problems and cardiovascular sickness. By advancing fat misfortune, especially in the stomach region,

irregular fasting can prompt a decrease in midriff circuit and upgrades in wellbeing.

6. Reasonable Weight reduction: Irregular fasting might offer a supportable way to deal with weight reduction and weight upkeep contrasted with customary calorie limitation eats fewer carbs. Since it doesn't need severe food limitations or steady calorie counting, discontinuous fasting can be more straightforward to stick to in the long haul, prompting supported weight reduction and further developed body creation. It's essential to note that singular outcomes might differ, and the viability of irregular fasting for weight reduction and body synthesis changes rely upon different elements, including diet quality, active work level, and way of life propensities. Irregular fasting may not be reasonable for everybody, and it's fundamental to talk with a medical services proficient or enrolled dietitian prior to beginning any fasting routine, particularly for people with basic ailments or explicit dietary necessities..

- Worked on Metabolic Wellbeing.

Discontinuous fasting (IF) has been displayed to work on different parts of metabolic wellbeing, prompting positive changes in markers, for example, insulin responsiveness, glucose control, and lipid profiles. This is the way irregular fasting can add to worked on metabolic wellbeing:

1. Insulin Responsiveness: Irregular fasting has been displayed to increment insulin awareness, which is the body's capacity to answer actually to insulin and control glucose levels. By diminishing insulin obstruction, irregular fasting can assist with bringing down fasting insulin levels and further develop glucose take-up by cells, prompting better glucose control and decreased chance of type 2 diabetes.

2. Glucose Control: Discontinuous fasting can prompt more steady glucose levels over the course of the day. By advancing glucose take-up by cells and decreasing glucose

creation by the liver, discontinuous fasting forestalls spikes and crashes in glucose levels, which might add to further developed energy levels, state of mind steadiness, and prosperity.

3. Lipid Profiles: Irregular fasting has been displayed to further develop lipid profiles by lessening levels of all out cholesterol, LDL cholesterol (frequently alluded to as "terrible" cholesterol), and fatty substances, while expanding levels of HDL cholesterol (frequently alluded to as "great" cholesterol). These progressions in lipid digestion are related to a lower chance of cardiovascular sickness and worked on cardiovascular wellbeing.

4. Irritation Decrease: Constant aggravation is a critical driver of metabolic brokenness and is ensnared in the improvement of heftiness, insulin obstruction, and other metabolic problems. Discontinuous fasting makes mitigating impacts, as proven by decreases in markers of irritation like C-receptive protein (CRP) and interleukin-6 (IL-6). By lessening persistent aggravation,

discontinuous fasting might assist with working on metabolic wellbeing and diminish the gamble of fiery infections.

5. Oxidative Pressure Decrease: Discontinuous fasting has been displayed to diminish oxidative pressure, which happens when there is an irregularity between free extremists and cancer prevention agents in the body. By upgrading cell reinforcement guards and advancing cell fix components, discontinuous fasting can assist with relieving oxidative harm to cells and tissues, which might add to worked on metabolic wellbeing and life span.

6. Mitochondrial Capability: Mitochondria are the energy-delivering organelles inside cells, and their brokenness is related to metabolic problems and maturing. Irregular fasting has been displayed to upgrade mitochondrial capability and biogenesis, prompting further developed energy creation, cell digestion, and metabolic wellbeing. Discontinuous fasting can significantly affect metabolic wellbeing by further developing insulin responsiveness,

glucose control, lipid profiles, aggravation, oxidative pressure, and mitochondrial capability. These metabolic enhancements add to a lower hazard of ongoing illnesses like sort 2 diabetes, cardiovascular sickness, and metabolic disorder, and may advance life span and prosperity.

- Mental Advantages and Mind Wellbeing.

Discontinuous fasting (IF) has been related to different mental advantages and enhancements in cerebrum wellbeing. This is the way irregular fasting can add to mental capability and cerebrum wellbeing:

1. Improved Cerebrum Inferred Neurotrophic Component (BDNF) Creation: Irregular fasting has been displayed to build the development of mind determined neurotrophic factor (BDNF), a protein that upholds the development, endurance, and capability of neurons. More elevated levels of BDNF are related with worked on mental capability, learning, and memory.

2. Brain adaptability: Discontinuous fasting advances brain adaptability, the mind's capacity to redesign and adjust considering encounters and natural changes. By animating the arrangement of new brain associations and synaptic pathways, irregular fasting might improve learning,

memory solidification, and mental adaptability.

3. Neuroprotection: Irregular fasting makes neuroprotective impacts, assisting with safeguarding neurons against oxidative pressure, irritation, and age-related harm. By lessening oxidative harm and advancing cell fix instruments, irregular fasting might assist with forestalling neurodegenerative illnesses, for example, Alzheimer's and Parkinson's sickness and defer age-related mental degradation.

4. Expanded Ketone Creation: During fasting periods, the body enters a condition of ketosis, where ketone bodies, for example, beta-hydroxybutyrate (BHB), are delivered as an elective fuel hotspot for the mind. Ketones are profoundly proficient energy substrates that give a consistent stock of fuel to the cerebrum, prompting worked on mental capability, mental clearness, and concentration.

5. Further developed Cerebrum Wellbeing Markers: Irregular fasting has been displayed to work on different markers of

mind wellbeing, including expanded mind inferred neurotrophic factor (BDNF) levels, diminished irritation, upgraded cell reinforcement protections, and improved mitochondrial capability. These progressions in cerebrum wellbeing markers are related with better mental capability, state of mind guideline, and generally mind flexibility.

6. Security Against Neurological Problems: Discontinuous fasting might help safeguard against age related neurological issues and mental degradation by advancing neurogenesis, diminishing oxidative pressure and irritation, and improving synaptic versatility. Arising research recommends that irregular fasting might have remedial potential for neurodegenerative sicknesses like Alzheimer's and Parkinson's infection. Discontinuous fasting offers promising mental advantages and may uphold mind wellbeing by advancing brain adaptability, neuroprotection, expanded ketone creation, and further developed cerebrum wellbeing markers. These impacts add to better mental

capability, mind-set guideline, and flexibility against age-related mental degradation and neurological problems. Notwithstanding, more examination is expected to completely grasp the system's basic discontinuous fasting consequences for mind wellbeing and to decide the ideal fasting regimens for boosting mental advantages.

Chapter Four
Carrying out Discontinuous Fasting.

Discontinuous fasting (IF) has been related to different mental advantages and upgrades in cerebrum wellbeing. This is the way irregular fasting can add to mental capability and cerebrum wellbeing:

1. Improved Mind Determined Neurotrophic Variable (BDNF) Creation: Discontinuous fasting has been displayed to build the development of cerebrum inferred neurotrophic factor (BDNF), a protein that upholds the development, endurance, and capability of neurons. More significant levels of BDNF are related to working on mental capability, learning, and memory.

2. Brain adaptability: Discontinuous fasting advances brain adaptability, the mind's capacity to redesign and adjust considering encounters and natural changes. By

invigorating the development of new brain associations and synaptic pathways, irregular fasting might improve learning, memory solidification, and mental adaptability.

3. Neuroprotection: Irregular fasting makes neuroprotective impacts, assisting with safeguarding neurons against oxidative pressure, irritation, and age-related harm. By lessening oxidative harm and advancing cell fix components, discontinuous fasting might assist with forestalling neurodegenerative sicknesses, for example, Alzheimer's and Parkinson's infection and defer age-related mental degradation.

4. Expanded Ketone Creation: During fasting periods, the body enters a condition of ketosis, where ketone bodies, for example, beta-hydroxybutyrate (BHB), are delivered as an elective fuel hotspot for the cerebrum. Ketones are exceptionally effective energy substrates that give a consistent inventory of fuel to the mind, prompting worked on mental capability, mental lucidity, and concentration.

5. Further developed Mind Wellbeing Markers: Intermittent fasting has been displayed to work on different markers of cerebrum wellbeing, including expanded mind inferred neurotrophic factor (BDNF) levels, diminished aggravation, upgraded cell reinforcement guards, and improved mitochondrial capability. These progressions in mind wellbeing markers are related with better mental capability, temperament guideline, and cerebrum strength.

6. Security Against Neurological Issues: Discontinuous fasting might help safeguard against age-related neurological problems and mental deterioration by advancing neurogenesis, decreasing oxidative pressure and aggravation, and improving synaptic pliancy. Arising research proposes that irregular fasting might have remedial potential for neurodegenerative illnesses like Alzheimer's and Parkinson's infection. Irregular fasting offers promising mental advantages and may uphold cerebrum wellbeing by advancing brain adaptability, neuroprotection, expanded ketone creation,

and further developed mind wellbeing markers. These impacts add to better mental capability, state of mind guideline, and versatility against age-related mental deterioration and neurological issues. More examination is expected to completely grasp the components hidden discontinuous fasting consequences for mind wellbeing and to decide the ideal fasting regimens for boosting mental advantages.

- Picking the Right Technique for You.

Picking the right discontinuous fasting (IF) technique for you relies upon different elements, including your way of life, inclinations, wellbeing objectives, and individual necessities. Here are a few contemplations to assist you with choosing the Assuming that strategy that adjusts best to your conditions:

1. Fasting Length: Consider how long you're happy with fasting and how it squeezes into your day to day everyday practice. Some if techniques include more limited fasting periods, for example, time-confined eating (e.g., 16/8 strategy), where you quick for 16 hours and eat inside an 8-hour window every day. Others, similar to substitute day fasting or intermittent fasting, may include longer fasting periods, going from 24 hours to a few days.

2. Recurrence of Fasting: Conclude how every now and again you're willing to be

quick. Some On the off chance that techniques require fasting consistently (e.g., time-confined eating), while others include fasting every other day (e.g., substitute day fasting) or occasionally (e.g., intermittent fasting). Pick a fasting recurrence that accommodates your way of life and considers adherence over the long haul.

3. Adaptability: Consider how adaptable you need your fasting timetable to be. Some if techniques offer greater adaptability in feast timing and fasting length, permitting you to change your fasting plan in view of your necessities and inclinations. Others might be more inflexible or organized, expecting adherence to explicit fasting and eating windows.

4. Dinner Timing: Assess when you like to eat your feasts and how it lines up with your everyday timetable and social responsibilities. Some On the off chance that techniques consider greater adaptability in dinner timing, while others have stricter rules on when to eat. Pick a technique that permits you to appreciate dinners

occasionally that are helpful and charming for you.

5. Wellbeing Contemplations: Consider any basic ailments or dietary limitations. Certain On the off chance that strategies may not be appropriate for everybody, particularly those with ailments like diabetes, dietary problems, or gastrointestinal issues. Talk with a medical services proficient or enrolled dietitian to decide whether on the off chance that is fitting for yourself and to fit a fasting routine to your singular necessities.

6. Long haul Maintainability: Evaluate the drawn out supportability of the In the event of that technique you decide. Consider whether it's something you can practically keep up with after some time and coordinate into your way of life as a reasonable dietary example. Search for a technique that advances wellbeing and prosperity and supports your wellbeing objectives over the long haul.

7. Individual Inclinations: At last, pick an assuming technique that resounds with your

own inclinations, values, and objectives. Try different things with various methodologies and pay attention to your body's input to find what turns out best for you. Recall that there is nobody size-fits-all the way to deal with IF, and it means a lot to fit your fasting routine to suit your singular necessities and inclinations. By considering these variables and picking the Assuming that technique that adjusts best to your way of life and objectives, you can expand the advantages of irregular fasting while partaking in a supportable and pleasant dietary example. Remain adaptable, pay attention to your body, and look for direction from a medical services proficient or enrolled dietitian if necessary.

- Tending to Normal Worries and misguided judgments.

Tending to normal worries and misguided judgments about irregular fasting (IF) can assist people with pursuing informed choices and have good expectations about consolidating IF into their way of life. Here are a few normal worries and misguided judgments about IF, alongside explanations:

1. Fasting Prompts Muscle Misfortune: One worry about Assuming is that it might prompt muscle misfortune because of broadened periods without food. Notwithstanding, research proposes that discontinuous fasting can save fit bulk, particularly when joined with opposition preparing and sufficient protein consumption. Fasting triggers hormonal changes that advance muscle protection and may try to improve muscle development after some time.

2. Fasting Dials Back Digestion: There is a misinterpretation that fasting dials back

digestion and prompts a reduction in energy use. While the metabolic rate may briefly diminish during fasting periods, studies have shown that irregular fasting doesn't adversely affect the metabolic rate in the long haul. As a matter of fact, IF can work on metabolic wellbeing by upgrading insulin responsiveness and advancing fat digestion.

3. Fasting Causes Supplement Lacks: Certain individuals stress that fasting might bring about supplement lacks because of decreased food consumption. Notwithstanding, discontinuous fasting can be viable with a reasonable and nutritious eating routine that gives fundamental nutrients, minerals, and micronutrients. By zeroing in on supplement thick food varieties during eating windows, people can meet their dietary necessities while fasting.

4. Fasting Is Risky for Specific Populaces: There is a misguided judgment that fasting is dangerous for specific populaces, for example, pregnant or breastfeeding ladies, people with diabetes, or those with a background marked by dietary problems.

While fasting may not be suitable for everybody, many people with legitimate direction and oversight securely drilled it. Talking with a medical care proficient or enrolled dietitian can help decide whether on the off chance that is reasonable for explicit conditions.

5. Fasting Prompts Voraciously consuming food: Certain individuals stress that fasting might set off gorging or scattered eating designs. While it's fundamental for approach fasting with care and mindfulness, research proposes that irregular fasting doesn't be guaranteed to prompt voraciously consuming food when polished dependably. Laying out a reasonable way to deal with eating during eating windows and tending to profound eating triggers can assist with forestalling gorging.

6. Fasting Is Just About Weight Loss: While discontinuous fasting is frequently connected with weight reduction, it offers a scope of medical advantages past weight the board. These advantages incorporate better metabolic wellbeing, improved mental

capability, expanded life span, and diminished hazard of persistent illnesses like sort 2 diabetes and cardiovascular sickness. Discontinuous fasting can advance prosperity and backing a sound way of life past weight reduction objectives. Tending to these normal worries and confusions can assist people with moving toward discontinuous fasting with certainty and come to informed conclusions about integrating it into their way of life. By understanding the likely advantages and contemplations of IF, people can fit their fasting routine to suit their singular necessities and inclinations while advancing wellbeing and prosperity.

- Useful Hints for Progress.

To prevail with discontinuous fasting (IF), consider executing the accompanying pragmatic tips:

1. Begin Gradually: if you're new to discontinuous fasting, slip into it slowly by continuously expanding fasting lengths or beginning with more limited fasting windows. This can assist your body with acclimating to the fasting routine all the more serenely.

2. Remain Hydrated: Drink a lot of water and other non-caloric refreshments during fasting periods to remain hydrated and check hunger. Home-grown tea, dark espresso, and shining water are great choices that can assist with smothering hunger.

3. Eat Supplement Thick Food sources: Spotlight on supplement thick food sources during eating windows to help wellbeing and prosperity. Incorporate various organic products, vegetables, lean proteins, sound fats, entire grains, and vegetables in your dinners to guarantee you're getting

fundamental nutrients, minerals, and supplements.

4. Plan Your Dinners: Plan your feasts and snacks early on to guarantee you have nutritious choices accessible during eating windows. Dinner preparing and clump preparing can assist with smoothing out feast planning and make smart dieting more helpful.

5. Stand by listening to Your Body: Focus on your body's yearning and satiety signs during fasting and eating periods. Eat when you're eager and stop when you're fulfilled. Try not to indulge or limiting food admission unreasonably and change your fasting routine case by case in view of your body's criticism.

6. Remain Occupied: Keep yourself involved and diverted during fasting periods to take your psyche off food desires. Take part in exercises like work, leisure activities, exercise, or associating to assist with relaxing and lessen the desire to eat.

7. Be Adaptable: Be adaptable with your fasting plan and consider changes depending

on the situation considering changes in your everyday practice, get-togethers, or unique events. It's OK to sometimes go amiss from your fasting routine, as long as you return to your normal timetable thereafter.

8. Screen Your Advancement: Monitor your advancement, remembering changes in weight, body piece, energy levels, and general prosperity. Observe any enhancements in metabolic wellbeing markers, for example, glucose levels, cholesterol levels, and pulse. Change your fasting routine case by case in view of your objectives and criticism from your body.

9. Look for Help: Find a steady local area or responsibility accomplice to share your discontinuous fasting venture with. Having consolation and backing from others can assist with keeping you inspired and focused on your fasting objectives.

10. Talk with an Expert: if you have any hidden medical issue or concerns, talk with a medical services proficient or enlisted dietitian prior to beginning discontinuous fasting. They can give customized direction

and proposals, considering your singular necessities and conditions. By integrating these functional tips into your discontinuous fasting schedule, you can get yourself in a good position and expand the advantages of IF for your wellbeing and prosperity. Move toward irregular fasting with care and mindfulness, and pay attention to your body's necessities in the interim.

Chapter Five
The Science Behind Appetite and Satiety.

Understanding the science behind craving and satiety is urgent for successfully overseeing food consumption and keeping a sound connection with eating. Here outlines the vital variables and components engaged with craving and satiety.

1. Hormonal Guideline: Craving and satiety are directed by an intricate transaction of chemicals and synapses that convey between the cerebrum, stomach, and different organs. Ghrelin, frequently alluded to as the "hunger chemical," animates craving and increments food consumption, while chemicals, for example, leptin, peptide YY (PYY), and cholecystokinin (CCK) signal satiety and lessen hunger.

2. Ghrelin: Delivered principally in the stomach, ghrelin levels increment before feasts and decline in the wake of eating. Ghrelin invigorates hunger by flagging the

mind to start food-chasing ways of behaving and increment food consumption. Elements affected levels of ghrelin, for example, dinner timing, macronutrient arrangement, and stress.

3. Leptin: Fat cells deliver Leptin and go about as a drawn out controller of energy balance by flagging the cerebrum to diminish food admission and increment energy consumption when fat stores are adequate. Leptin opposition, where the cerebrum turns out to be less receptive to leptin signals, can add to indulging and stoutness.

4. Peptide YY (PYY) and Cholecystokinin (CCK): Delivered in the gastrointestinal parcel because of food admission, PYY and CCK assist with advancing satiety by easing back gastric discharging, lessening craving, and upgrading sensations of completion. These chemicals assume a part in controlling dinner size and recurrence.

5. Insulin and Glucose Levels: Insulin, a chemical delivered by the pancreas because of food consumption, directs glucose levels

and works with the take-up of glucose into cells for energy. Variances in glucose levels can impact appetite and satiety, with fast spikes and drops in glucose adding to expanded yearning and desires.

6. Brain Flagging: Brain signals from the stomach and different organs speak with the mind to direct hunger and food consumption. Tactile signals like taste, smell, and surface of food, as well as mental and close to home elements, can likewise impact yearning and satiety prompts.

7. Stomach Microbiota: Arising research recommends that the stomach microbiota, the different local area of microorganisms in the gastrointestinal plot, may assume a part in craving guideline and energy digestion. Certain stomach microscopic organisms produce metabolites that impact appetite and satiety flags and may influence food inclinations and desires. Understanding the science behind appetite and satiety can assist people with settling on informed decisions about their dietary patterns, including dinner timing, segment control, and food choice.

By focusing on yearning and satiety prompts, adjusting hormonal signals, and embracing careful eating rehearses, people can advance ideal craving guideline and keep a solid relationship with food.

- Understanding Appetite Signs.

Understanding craving signals is fundamental for successfully overseeing food consumption and advancing a solid relationship with eating. Here are a few critical parts of yearning signs to consider:

1. Physiological Yearning: Physiological craving is the body's normal reaction to a requirement for energy and supplements. Actual sensations regularly described it, for example, stomach snarling, low energy levels, and a craving to eat. Physiological appetite signals are directed by hormonal and brain systems that are impart of the mind, stomach, and different organs.

2. Ghrelin Delivery: Ghrelin is frequently alluded to as the "hunger chemical" since it animates craving and advances food consumption. Ghrelin levels commonly increment before dinners and diminishing after eating, flagging craving and satiety in the mind. Vacillations in ghrelin levels are impacted by elements, for example, dinner

timing, macronutrient arrangement, and stress.

3. Low Glucose: Low glucose levels, otherwise called hypoglycemia, can set off hunger signals as the body tries to renew glucose stores and keep up with energy balance. Fast drops in glucose levels, frequently connected with skipping dinners or eating high-sugar food varieties, can prompt expanded sensations of appetite and desires.

4. Stomach Compressions: Food cravings or stomach constrictions are a typical actual sensation related to hunger. These withdrawals happen when the stomach is vacant and animate ghrelin, flagging craving to the mind. Eating ordinary feasts and bites can assist with forestalling extreme stomach constrictions and oversee hunger levels.

5. Time Since Last Dinner: The time since your last feast can impact hunger signals. Over the long haul, without food admission, hunger regularly increments, flagging the body's requirement for sustenance. Irregular fasting regimens that include delayed fasting

periods might prompt elevated hunger signals during fasting windows.

6. Hydration Status: Parchedness can sometimes be confused with hunger, as thirst signs might be misconstrued as a requirement for food. Drinking water or other non-caloric refreshments can assist with extinguishing thirst and lessen sensations of craving. Remaining hydrated over the course of the day can assist with keeping up with ideal hydration status and forestall superfluous nibbling.

7. Mind-Body Association: Profound and mental elements can likewise impact hunger signals. Stress, fatigue, forlornness, uneasiness, and different feelings might set off desires and the longing to eat, even without a trace of actual yearning. Rehearsing care and profound mindfulness can assist with recognizing genuine appetite and close to home eating triggers. By understanding yearning signals and the variables that impact them, people can foster procedures to oversee hunger, forestall gorging, and advance careful dietary

patterns. Paying attention to your body's signals, eating normal dinners and bites, remaining hydrated, and closing to home eating triggers can assist encourage a sound connection with food and backing prosperity.

- The Job of Ghrelin and Leptin.

Ghrelin and leptin are two key chemicals associated with the guideline of craving and satiety, assuming correlative parts in keeping up with energy balance and controlling food admission. Here outlines the jobs of ghrelin and leptin: Ghrelin:

1. Hunger Chemical: Ghrelin, frequently alluded to as the "hunger chemical," is basically created in the stomach and delivered into the circulatory system because of void stomach conditions and low energy accessibility.

2. Animates Hunger: Ghrelin animates craving and advances food consumption by following up on receptors in the nerve center and other mind areas engaged with craving guideline. It increments hunger sensations, triggers food-chasing ways of behaving, and upgrades the remunerating properties of food.

3. Guideline of Dinner Commencement: Ghrelin levels commonly ascend before feasts and pinnacle not long prior to eating,

flagging craving and advancing dinner inception. After food consumption, ghrelin levels decline, adding to sensations of satiety and lessening the drive to eat.

4. Impact of Variables: different elements affect Ghrelin levels, including feast timing, macronutrient structure, stress, rest designs, and circadian rhythms. Variances in ghrelin levels assist with managing hunger and energy balance considering changes in dietary and ecological circumstances.

Leptin:

1. Satiety Chemical: Leptin, created essentially by fat cells (adipocytes), goes about as a drawn out controller of energy equilibrium and body weight by flagging satiety and diminishing food consumption.

2. Guideline of Fat Stores: Leptin levels are corresponding to muscle versus fat stores, with more elevated levels emitted in people with more noteworthy fat mass. Leptin signals the cerebrum to diminish appetite and increment energy consumption when fat

stores are adequate, assisting with keeping up with energy balance and forestall overabundance weight gain.

3. Criticism System: Leptin follows up on receptors in the nerve center and other cerebrum districts to control hunger and energy consumption. It gives input to the mind about energy status and supplement accessibility, assisting with planning metabolic cycles and change food admission appropriately.

4. Leptin Opposition: now and again of heftiness, people might create leptin obstruction, where the mind turns out to be less receptive to leptin signals notwithstanding raised leptin levels. Leptin obstruction can disturb hunger guideline and add to indulging and weight gain.

Ghrelin and leptin assume corresponding parts in managing yearning and satiety, with ghrelin animating craving and advancing food admission, while leptin signals satiety and lessens hunger. The harmony between these chemicals keeps up with energy equilibrium and control food consumption, adding to metabolic wellbeing and body weight guideline.

- Mental Parts of Eating Conduct.

The mental parts of eating conduct assume a huge part in molding our relationship with food, impacting food decisions, eating examples, and generally speaking, dietary propensities. Here are a few key mental variables that impact eating conduct:

1. Feelings: Feelings can capably affect eating conduct, prompting both gorging and undereating because of various profound states. Stress, tension, bitterness, weariness, satisfaction, and dejection are among the feelings that can impact food consumption. Profound eating, where people use food to adapt to or lighten close to home trouble, is a typical peculiarity that can add to unfortunate eating examples and weight gain.

2. Social Impacts: Social elements, including social standards, relational peculiarities, peer pressure, parties, and media impacts, assume a critical part in

forming eating conduct. Social eating ways of behaving, for example, eating because of meaningful gestures or friend pressure, can influence food decisions and peace sizes. Social conditions that advance unfortunate dietary patterns or food signs can add to indulging and undesirable dietary examples.

3. Food Inclinations and Desires: Individual food inclinations and desires are impacted by a mix of hereditary, ecological, and mental variables. Taste inclinations, previous encounters with food, openness to food publicizing, and a learned relationship among food and award can shape food decisions and utilization designs. Desires for explicit food sources, especially those high in sugar, fat, or salt, can be driven by physiological elements, profound signals, or change.

4. Careful Eating: Careful eating includes focusing on the tangible experience of eating, including taste, surface, smell, and actual yearning signals, without judgment or interruption. Careful eating practices can assist people with fostering a more

noteworthy consciousness of their dietary patterns, further develop segment control, and encourage a more sure relationship with food. By tuning into yearning and satiety prompts and relishing each nibble, people can advance better eating ways of behaving and decrease careless or profound eating.

5. Mental Elements: Mental variables, like convictions, perspectives, discernments, and self-administrative cycles, additionally impact eating conduct. Mental cycles connected with food decision, segment control, restraint, and food-related navigation can affect dietary propensities and weight the board results. Mental rebuilding strategies, for example, testing negative considerations about food or self-perception, can assist people with creating better eating ways of behaving and perspectives.

6. Dietary issues: Dietary issues, for example, anorexia nervosa, bulimia nervosa, and pigging out jumble, include complex associations between mental, organic, and ecological elements. Twisted self-

perception, feeling of dread toward weight gain, low confidence, compulsiveness, and injury are among the mental variables related to dietary issues. Treatment approaches for dietary issues normally address both the mental and social parts of confused eating ways of behaving. Understanding the mental parts of eating conduct can assist people with creating systems to advance better dietary patterns, deal with close to home eating triggers, and cultivate a positive relationship with food. By tending to fundamental mental factors and taking on careful eating rehearses, people can roll out practical improvements to their dietary propensities and, in general, prosperity.

Chapter Six
Expected Dangers and Contemplations.

While irregular fasting (IF) can offer different medical advantages for some people, there are additionally likely dangers and contemplations to know about. Here are a few elements to consider:

1. Wholesome Inadequacies: Contingent upon the particular fasting routine followed and dietary decisions made during eating windows, there is a gamble of lacking supplement consumption. Delayed fasting periods or prohibitive eating examples might prompt lacks in fundamental supplements like nutrients, minerals, and macronutrients. It's vital to focus on supplement thick food sources and guarantee a decent eating regimen to relieve this gamble.

2. Disarranged Eating Examples: Irregular fasting might fuel or set off scattered eating ways of behaving in defenseless people, especially those with a background marked

by dietary problems or an inclination to prohibitive eating designs. Checking for indications of over the top contemplations about food, unnecessary calorie limitation, or sensations of culpability or disgrace connected with eating is pivotal, and looking for proficient help might be vital if confused eating ways of behaving arise.

3. Influence on Digestion: While discontinuous fasting can work on metabolic wellbeing for some people, it may not be appropriate for everybody, especially those with fundamental metabolic circumstances like diabetes or hypoglycemia. Fasting can influence glucose levels, insulin responsiveness, and metabolic rate, and people with metabolic issues ought to talk with a medical services proficient prior to beginning an IF routine.

4. Potential for Muscle Misfortune: Expanded fasting periods or deficient protein admission during eating windows might build the gamble of muscle misfortune, especially for people who are truly dynamic or take part in strength

preparing. It's fundamental to focus on protein-rich food sources and opposition exercise to help muscle support and forestall loss of fit weight.

5. Influence on Hormonal Equilibrium: Irregular fasting can impact hormonal equilibrium, remembering changes for cortisol, thyroid chemicals, and conceptive chemicals. While certain people might encounter hormonal transformations that help metabolic wellbeing and fat misfortune, others might be more delicate to disturbances in hormonal equilibrium. Checking for indications of hormonal uneven characters, for example, sporadic monthly cycles or changes in temperament and energy levels, is significant, and talking with a medical care proficient might be important if concerns emerge.

6. Potential for Indulging: Following times of fasting, there might be a propensity to gorge or consume bigger parts during eating windows, which can invalidate the calorie shortage made by fasting. Rehearsing careful eating, focusing on craving and

satiety prompts, and zeroing in on supplement thick food varieties can assist with forestalling gorging and elevate a fair way to deal with eating.

7. Individual Inconstancy: It's critical to perceive that singular reactions to discontinuous fasting can shift broadly. Factors like age, sex, hereditary qualities, way of life, and hidden medical issue can impact the viability and security of IF for various people. It's fundamental to pay attention to your body, screen your reaction to fasting, and change your method depending on the situation in view of your one of a kind necessities and conditions. While irregular fasting can offer advantages for certain people, it's vital to move toward it carefully and think about dangers and contemplations. Talking with a medical care proficient or enlisted dietitian prior to beginning and On the off chance that routine can assist with guaranteeing that it's protected and proper for you, especially assuming that you have hidden ailments or worries about what fasting might mean for

your wellbeing. Also, rehearsing control, equilibrium, and adaptability in your way to deal with fasting can assist with advancing prosperity and reasonable dietary propensities.

- Influence on Bulk.

Discontinuous fasting (IF) may influence bulk contingent upon different factors, like fasting span, dietary protein admission, practice routine, and individual digestion. This is the way IF can influence bulk:

1. Protein Admission: Satisfactory protein admission is fundamental for safeguarding bulk, particularly during times of fasting. Consuming adequate protein during eating windows can assist with supporting muscle upkeep and fix during fasting periods. Counting protein-rich food sources like lean meats, poultry, fish, eggs, dairy items, vegetables, and tofu in feasts can assist with addressing protein needs and moderate the gamble of muscle misfortune.

2. Obstruction Exercise: taking part in opposition preparing or strength preparing activities can assist safeguard and work with muscling mass while following a discontinuous fasting routine. Opposition

practice animates muscle protein combination and advances muscle development, assisting with neutralizing any potential muscle misfortune related to fasting. Integrating normal strength instructional meetings into your work-out routine can assist with keeping up with bulk and backing body organization objectives.

3. Fasting Length: The term and recurrence of fasting periods can impact their effect on bulk. More limited fasting terms, for example, those related to time-confined eating (e.g., 16/8 strategy), may insignificantly affect bulk, especially when joined with sufficient protein admission and obstruction work out. Delayed fasting periods or more prohibitive fasting regimens might build the gamble in muscle misfortune, particularly assuming protein admission is deficient.

4. Hormonal Changes: Irregular fasting can influence chemical levels, including insulin, development chemical, and cortisol, which can impact muscle digestion and protein combination. While fasting may at first lead

to an expansion in cortisol levels, which can advance muscle breakdown, the general effect on bulk relies upon variables like protein admission, exercise, and individual reactions to fasting.

5. Individual Inconstancy: Individual reactions to irregular fasting can shift for certain people encountering more prominent muscle protection or even muscle development during fasting periods, while others might be more helpless to muscle misfortune. Factors like age, sex, hereditary qualities, digestion, and eating regimen and way of life propensities can impact how the body answers fasting as far as bulk changes. In outline, discontinuous fasting can affect bulk contingent upon different variables, including protein consumption, work out, fasting span, and individual changeability. To limit the gamble of muscle misfortune and backing muscle upkeep while following and In the event of that routine, it's critical to focus on sufficient protein consumption, take part in normal opposition exercise, and screen your body's reaction to fasting.

Talking with a medical care proficient or enrolled dietitian can give customized direction to enhancing bulk while rehearsing discontinuous fasting.

- Consequences for Athletic Execution.

Discontinuous fasting (IF) can meaningfully affect athletic execution, contingent upon variables like the fasting term, timing of activity, supplement admission, and individual reactions. This is a breakdown of the way IF may influence athletic execution: Constructive outcomes:

1. Body Organization: A few investigations recommend that irregular fasting can advance fat misfortune while protecting slender bulk, which might help competitors meaning to further develop body creation and decrease muscle to fat ratio.

2. Metabolic Variations: Irregular fasting can prompt metabolic transformations, for example, expanded fat oxidation and further developed insulin responsiveness, which might improve perseverance execution and metabolic productivity during exercise.

3. Upgraded Recuperation: Irregular fasting might advance cell fix instruments, for

example, autophagy, which might actually improve recuperation from work out incited muscle harm and decrease aggravation.

4. Accommodation: For certain competitors, discontinuous fasting might offer comfort and adaptability in feast timing, permitting them to plan instructional meetings and contests around fasting and eating windows.

Adverse consequences:

1. Diminished Energy Availability: Fasting periods can bring about diminished energy accessibility, which might debilitate practice execution, especially extreme focus or delayed perseverance exercises that require glycogen stores for fuel.

2. Muscle Misfortune: Expanded fasting periods or lacking protein consumption during eating windows might build the gamble of muscle misfortune, which can adversely influence strength, influence, and muscle perseverance.

3. Weariness and Laziness: A few people might encounter weakness, torpidity, or

decreased energy levels during fasting periods, which can debilitate inspiration, concentration, and exercise execution.

4. Hydration Status: Fasting can influence hydration status, particularly during fasting periods that correspond to instructional courses or rivalries. Insufficient liquid admission might prompt lack of hydration, which can disable mental capability, thermoregulation, and exercise execution.

Contemplations for Competitors:

1.   Individualization:The impacts of discontinuous fasting on athletic execution change among people, and what works for one competitor may not work for another. It's fundamental for competitors to explore different avenues regarding different fasting regimens, screen their presentation and recuperation, and change their method considering individual reactions.

2. Timing of Eating and Preparing: Timing feasts and instructional meetings decisively

can assist with improving athletic execution while rehearsing discontinuous fasting. Consuming sugars and protein when exercises can uphold energy levels, muscle glycogen recharging, and muscle recuperation.

3. Hydration and Electrolytes: Competitors ought to focus on hydration and electrolyte balance, especially during fasting periods and extreme instructional meetings. Devouring liquids and electrolyte-rich food varieties during eating windows can assist with keeping up with hydration status and backing exercise execution.

4. Interview with Experts: Competitors considering irregular fasting ought to talk with a medical care proficient, enlisted dietitian, or sports nutritionist to guarantee that their nourishing requirements are met, and their fasting routine is viable with their preparation and execution objectives. Taking everything into account, irregular fasting can affect athletic execution, and its effect shifts among people. Competitors ought to painstakingly think about the

advantages and dangers of irregular fasting, explore different avenues regarding different fasting regimens, and focus on sustenance, hydration, and recuperation to help their preparation and execution objectives.

- Wellbeing Worries for Specific Populaces.

Discontinuous fasting (IF) may not be reasonable for specific populaces, and there are explicit wellbeing worries to consider for people with specific medical issue or conditions. Here are a few gatherings for whom discontinuous fasting may not be suitable or require cautious thought:

1. Pregnant or Breastfeeding Ladies: Pregnant or breastfeeding ladies have expanded energy and supplement needs to help fetal development, lactation, and maternal wellbeing. Discontinuous fasting may not give sufficient energy or supplements during pivotal phases of pregnancy or breastfeeding and might actually adversely influence maternal and fetal wellbeing. Pregnant or breastfeeding ladies ought to focus on offset nourishment and talk with a medical services proficient

prior to thinking about discontinuous fasting.

2. Youngsters and Teenagers: Kids and youths have remarkable wholesome prerequisites for development, improvement, and wellbeing. Irregular fasting might impede development and advancement by limiting fundamental supplements and calories during basic times of development. Executing fasting regimens in this populace ought to be drawn closer with alert and under the direction of a medical services proficient.

3. People with Dietary issues: People with a background marked by dietary problems or confused eating examples might be especially defenseless against the prohibitive idea of irregular fasting and might be in danger of compounding disarranged eating ways of behaving. Fasting regimens can set off sensations of culpability, disgrace, or tension around food and self-perception, possibly prompting unfortunate associations with food and negative mental results. People with dietary problems or a

background marked by cluttered eating ought to keep away from discontinuous fasting and look for fitting treatment and backing.

4. Underweight People: Underweight people, incorporating those with a low weight record (BMI) or history of hunger, might be in danger of additional supplement lacks and compromised wellbeing results in discontinuous fasting. Fasting could fuel insufficient calorie admission and supplement retention, prompting further weight reduction, muscle squandering, and supplement inadequacies. Underweight people really must focus on standard feasts and snacks to help weight gain and wellbeing.

5. People with diabetes: People with diabetes, especially type 1 diabetes or insulin-subordinate sort 2 diabetes, ought to move toward irregular fasting with alert and under the direction of a medical care proficient. Fasting can influence glucose levels and insulin awareness, possibly prompting hypoglycemia or hyperglycemia.

Close checking of glucose levels, changes under prescription measurements, and cautious administration of fasting and eating windows are important to guarantee security and advance glycemic control.

6. People with Constant Medical issue: People with persistent ailments like cardiovascular infection, kidney illness, liver sickness, or immune system problems might have explicit dietary requirements and limitations that irregular fasting could affect. Fasting might influence prescription digestion, pulse, electrolyte balance, and other physiological boundaries, possibly compounding basic medical issue. It's fundamental for people with persistent medical issue to talk with a medical care proficient prior to beginning discontinuous fasting and to screen their wellbeing status throughout the fasting routine intently.

7. More established Grown-ups: More established grown-ups may have different wholesome necessities and metabolic reactions to fasting contrasted with more youthful people. Fasting could compound

age-related muscle misfortune, sarcopenia, or mental deterioration in more seasoned grown-ups, especially if satisfactory protein admission and muscle-reinforcing exercise are not kept up with. More seasoned grown-ups ought to focus on adjusted sustenance and think about the expected effect of fasting on their general wellbeing and prosperity. In rundown, irregular fasting may not be fitting for specific populaces, including pregnant or breastfeeding ladies, kids and youths, people with dietary issues, underweight people, those with diabetes or constant ailments, and more seasoned grown ups. It's significant for people considering discontinuous fasting to talk with a medical services proficient or enlisted dietitian to evaluate their singular conditions, nourishing requirements, and expected takes a chance prior to beginning a fasting routine. Also, close observing of wellbeing status and changes under the fasting routine might be important to guarantee security and upgrade wellbeing results for these populaces.

Chapter Seven
Joining Discontinuous Fasting with Other Way of life Elements.

Joining irregular fasting (IF) with other way of life elements can improve its adequacy and advance wellbeing and prosperity. Here are some way of life variables to think about incorporating with discontinuous fasting:

1. Sound Eating routine: Matching irregular fasting with a reasonable and nutritious eating routine can upgrade wellbeing results and backing weight the executives objectives. Center on devouring entire, supplement thick food sources like organic products, vegetables, lean proteins, entire grains, and solid fats during eating windows. Focus on supplement rich feasts that give fundamental nutrients, minerals, and macronutrients to fuel your body and backing metabolic wellbeing.

2. Customary Actual work: Integrating normal actual work into your routine can

supplement discontinuous fasting by advancing fat misfortune, protecting fit bulk, and working on wellness. Take part in a mix of high-impact workout, strength preparing, and adaptability activities to help cardiovascular wellbeing, muscle strength, and portability. Go for the gold 150 minutes of moderate-power oxygen consuming action or 75 minutes of vivacious power vigorous action each week, alongside muscle-reinforcing exercises on at least two days out of every week.

3. Sufficient Hydration: Remaining hydrated is fundamental for wellbeing and prosperity, especially during fasting periods. Drink a lot of water and other hydrating liquids over the course of the day, particularly during eating windows, to keep up with ideal hydration status. Hydration upholds assimilation, supplement retention, metabolic capability, and cell hydration, assisting with advancing wellbeing and energy levels.

4. Quality Rest: Focus on quality rest as a feature of your discontinuous fasting way of life, as sufficient rest is critical for metabolic

wellbeing, chemical guideline, and prosperity. Hold back nothing long stretches of helpful rest each evening and lay out a reliable rest timetable to help circadian rhythms and enhance rest quality. Make a loosening up sleep time schedule, limit screen time before bed, and establish an agreeable rest climate to advance peaceful rest.

5. Stress The board: Persistent pressure can adversely affect wellbeing and upset metabolic cycles, possibly subverting the advantages of irregular fasting. Integrate pressure the executives methods like care reflection, profound breathing activities, yoga, kendo, or moderate muscle unwinding into your everyday daily practice to advance unwinding, lessen feelings of anxiety, and backing prosperity.

6. Social Help: Encircle yourself with a strong informal community that urges and spurs you to keep up with your discontinuous fasting routine and other solid way of life propensities. Share your objectives, difficulties, and triumphs with

companions, relatives, or online networks who can give consolation, responsibility, and useful help along your excursion.

7. Customary Wellbeing Observing: Routinely screen your wellbeing boundaries, including weight, body peace, circulatory strain, glucose levels, cholesterol levels, and other pertinent markers. Keeping tabs on your development can assist you with surveying the adequacy of your irregular fasting routine and recognize any potential wellbeing concerns or regions for development. Talk with a medical services proficient or enrolled dietitian if you have any different feedback about your wellbeing status or fasting routine. By incorporating this way of life factors with discontinuous fasting, you can improve the advantages of IF and advance wellbeing, prosperity, and life span. Try different things with various blends of way of life elements to find what turns out best for yourself and supports your singular wellbeing and health objectives.

- Practice and Active work Proposals.

Integrating exercise and actual work into your routine is fundamental for supporting wellbeing, upgrading wellness levels, and supplementing irregular fasting. Here are a few activity and active work suggestions to consider:

1. Vigorous Activity: Remember standard high-impact practice for your daily schedule to work on cardiovascular wellbeing, perseverance, and calorie use. Go for the gold 150 minutes of moderate-power high-impact action (like lively strolling, cycling, swimming, or moving) or 75 minutes of incredible force oxygen consuming movement (like running, HIIT exercises, or vigorous classes) each week. Separate your activity meetings into reasonable additions throughout the week to meet these proposals.

2. Strength Preparing: Integrate obstruction preparing or strength preparing practices into your daily schedule to assemble and

keep up with bulk, further develop strength, and backing metabolic wellbeing. Incorporate activities that target significant muscle gatherings, like squats, lurches, deadlifts, chest presses, lines, and shoulder presses. Expect to perform strength preparing practices no less than two days out of every week, with an emphasis on moderate over-burden to ceaselessly challenge your muscles and advance development.

3. Adaptability and Versatility: Remember to incorporate adaptability and portability practices in your daily schedule to work on the joint scope of movement, forestall wounds, and upgrade versatility and useful development. Consolidate extending practices for significant muscle gatherings, as well as exercises like yoga, Pilates, or judo, which center on adaptability, equilibrium, and body mindfulness. Mean to incorporate adaptability practices on most days of the week to keep up with and work on joint adaptability and versatility.

4. Span Preparing: Consider integrating stretch preparation or stop and go aerobic exercise (HIIT) exercises into your daily schedule to help calorie consume, work on cardiovascular wellness, and improve metabolic capability. Stretch preparation includes shifting back and forth between times of focused energy exercise and recuperation or lower-force movement. These exercises can be performed with different oxygen consuming activity, like running, cycling, or bodyweight works out, and can be adjusted to your wellness level and inclinations.

5. Dynamic Way of life: Search for valuable chances to integrate actual work into your day to day routine by taking on a functioning way of life. Use the stairwell rather than the lift, walk or bicycle for transportation whenever the situation allows, stand or move around during stationary exercises, and take part in sporting exercises or leisure activities that include development. All of the actual work adds up and adds to wellbeing and prosperity.

6. Stand by listening to Your Body: Focus on your body's signals and change your work-out daily schedule depending on the situation in view of how you feel. Assuming you're encountering weariness, irritation, or different indications of over training, permit yourself sufficient rest and recuperation time to forestall injury and advance execution. Be aware of any progressions in energy levels, mind-set, or actual side effects, and talk with a medical services proficient on the off chance that you have any worries or inquiries concerning your activity routine.

7. Remain Hydrated and Fuel Appropriately: Hydration and legitimate sustenance are fundamental for supporting activity execution, recuperation, and in general, wellbeing. Drink a lot of water previously, during, and after exercise to remain hydrated, and consider polishing off a fair feast or tidbit that incorporates sugars and protein to fuel your exercises and backing muscle recuperation. Be aware of your supplement and calorie needs, particularly while consolidating discontinuous fasting

with work out, and change your eating designs in like manner to help your movement levels and execution objectives. By integrating an assortment of oxygen consuming, strength, adaptability, and stretch preparation practices into your daily schedule and keeping a functioning way of life, you can expand the advantages of irregular fasting and backing wellbeing, wellness, and prosperity. Pay attention to your body, remain hydrated, and fuel appropriately to enhance your activity execution and recuperation.

- Nourishing Contemplations and Dinner Arranging.

Healthful contemplations and dinner arranging are pivotal parts of an effective discontinuous fasting (IF) routine. Here are a few hints to assist you with upgrading your sustenance and plan your feasts really while rehearsing irregular fasting:

1. Center on Supplement Thick Food sources: Focus on supplement thick food varieties that give fundamental nutrients, minerals, cell reinforcements, and macronutrients to help wellbeing and prosperity. Incorporate different natural products, vegetables, lean proteins, entire grains, solid fats, and vegetables in your dinners to guarantee you're meeting your supplement needs during eating windows.

2. Adjusted Feasts: Intend to make adjusted dinners that contain a mix of sugars, protein, and sound fats to help satiety, energy levels, and metabolic wellbeing. Integrate a

wellspring of lean protein (like poultry, fish, tofu, beans, or Greek yogurt), complex carbs (like entire grains, natural products, and vegetables), and sound fats (like nuts, seeds, avocado, or olive oil) into every dinner to advance supplement equilibrium and fulfillment.

3. Dinner Timing: Plan your feasts decisively to match with your fasting and eating windows and to help your energy needs over the course of the day. Consider timing your bigger feasts or higher-sugar dinners around times of expanded action or exercise to improve energy levels and execution. Try different things with various feast timing procedures to find what turns out best for your timetable and inclinations.

4. Hydration: Remain hydrated over the course of the day by drinking a lot of water and other hydrating liquids during both fasting and eating windows. Expect to drink somewhere around 8-10 cups of water each day, or more assuming you're genuinely dynamic or in blistering climate. Hydration upholds processing, supplement retention,

metabolic capability, and wellbeing, so focus on satisfactory liquid admission as a feature of your dinner arranging.

5. Pre-and Post-Exercise Nourishment: Consider your pre-and post-exercise sustenance needs while arranging your feasts around practice meetings. Consume a fair dinner or bite that incorporates sugars and protein before exercises to fuel your activity execution and backing muscle glycogen renewal. After exercises, focus on a mix of sugars and protein to help muscle recuperation and fix.

6. Segment Control: Focus on segment sizes and practice careful eating to forestall gorging during eating windows. Use obvious signs, segment control apparatuses, or estimating cups to assist you with checking fitting piece sizes for various food sources. Center on eating gradually, biting your food completely, and tuning into appetite and satiety signals to forestall extreme calorie admission and advance fulfillment.

7. Feast Variety: Integrate different food varieties and flavors into your dinners to

keep them fascinating and charming. Try different things with various foods, cooking strategies, and recipes to change up your eating routine and forestall weariness from your dinners. Incorporate a rainbow of beautiful leafy foods, spices and flavors, entire grains, and plant-based proteins to make tasty and nutritious dinners.

8. Prepare: Plan your feasts and snacks ahead of time to guarantee you have nutritious choices accessible during eating windows and to try not to depend on accommodation or cheap food choices. Consider bunch preparing or feast preparing fixings ahead of time to save time during the week and make it more straightforward to rapidly gather adjusted dinners. By considering these wholesome contemplations and feast arranging techniques, you can improve your nourishment, support your discontinuous fasting routine, and advance wellbeing and prosperity. Stand by listening to your body, focus on supplement thick food sources, and find a dinner arranging approach that turns

out best for your way of life and inclinations.

-Week by week feast plan, recipe and bit by bit directions on the most proficient method to make the recipe's.

Sure! Here is an example week by week feast plan with recipes and bit by bit directions for every recipe:

Day 1: Breakfast - Avocado Toast with Poached Eggs.

Ingredients:
- 2 cuts of entire grain bread
 - 1 ready avocado
- 2 eggs
- Salt and pepper to taste
- Discretionary fixings: cherry tomatoes, red pepper drops, or feta cheddar.

Instructions:

1. Toast the entire grain bread cuts until brilliant brown.

2. While the bread is toasting, set up the poached eggs. Carry a pot of water to a stew, then add a sprinkle of vinegar. Break each egg into a little bowl and delicately slide them into the stewing water. Poach the eggs for around 3-4 minutes until the whites are set yet the yolks are as yet runny.

3. Squash the ready avocado in a bowl and season with salt and pepper.

4. Spread the pounded avocado uniformly onto the toasted bread cuts.

5. Use an opened spoon to eliminate the poached eggs from the water and put them on top of the avocado toast.

6. Embellish with discretionary garnishes, for example, cut cherry tomatoes, red pepper chips, or disintegrated feta cheddar, whenever wanted.

7. Serve right away and appreciate!

Day1: Lunch - Quinoa Salad with Chickpeas and Vegetables:

Ingredients:
- 1 cup cooked quinoa
- 1 cup canned chickpeas, depleted and flushed - 1 cucumber, diced
- 1 chime pepper, diced
- 1/2 red onion, finely slashed
- 1/4 cup new parsley, cleaved
- Juice of 1 lemon
- 2 tablespoons olive oil
- Salt and pepper to taste

Instructions:
1. In an enormous blending bowl, join the cooked quinoa, chickpeas, diced cucumber, diced chime pepper, hacked red onion, and cleaved parsley.
2. In a little bowl, whisk together the lemon juice, olive oil, salt, and pepper to make the dressing.
3. Pour the dressing over the quinoa salad and prepare until very much merged.

4. Change preparing to taste, adding more salt, pepper, or lemon juice whenever wanted.

5. Partition the quinoa salad into individual serving bowls and trimming with extra parsley, whenever wanted.

6. Serve chilled or at room temperature and appreciate!

Day 1: Supper - Heated Salmon with Cooked Vegetables:

Ingredients:
- 2 salmon filets
- 2 tablespoons olive oil
- 2 cloves garlic, minced
- 1 teaspoon dried thyme
- 1 teaspoon paprika
- Salt and pepper to taste
- 2 cups blended vegetables (like broccoli, carrots, and chime peppers), cleaved
- Lemon wedges for serving

Instructions:

1. Preheat the stove to 400°F (200°C). Line a baking sheet with material paper.

2. Put the salmon filets on the pre-arranged baking sheet. Shower with olive oil and sprinkle with minced garlic, dried thyme, paprika, salt, and pepper.

3. Throw the slashed vegetables with olive oil, salt, and pepper on another baking sheet.

4. Place both the salmon and vegetables in the preheated stove and prepare for 15-20 minutes, or until the salmon is cooked through and the vegetables are delicate and softly sauteed.

5. Eliminate from the broiler and let cool somewhat prior to serving.

6. Serve the heated salmon with broiled vegetables close by lemon wedges for crushing over the fish.

7. Partake in your nutritious and scrumptious supper!

Day 2 : Breakfast - Greek Yogurt Parfait:

Ingredients:
- 1 cup Greek yogurt
- 1/2 cup blended berries (like strawberries, blueberries, and raspberries)
- 1/4 cup granola
- 1 tablespoon honey or maple syrup (discretionary)
- Discretionary garnishes: cut almonds, destroyed coconut, or chia seeds

Instructions:
1. In a serving glass or bowl, later Greek yogurt, blended berries, and granola.
2. Shower honey or maple syrup over the parfait, whenever wanted, for added pleasantness.
3. Rehash the layering system until the glass or bowl is filled, finishing with a sprinkle of granola on top.
4. Decorate with discretionary fixings like cut almonds, destroyed coconut, or chia seeds, whenever wanted.

5. Serve right away and partake in your reviving and nutritious parfait!

Day 2: Lunch - Turkey and Hummus Wrap:

Ingredients:
- 1 entire wheat tortilla or wrap
- 2-3 cuts of store turkey bosom
- 2 tablespoons hummus
- 1/4 cup blended greens (like spinach or lettuce)
- 1/4 cup destroyed carrots
- 1/4 avocado, cut (discretionary)
- Salt and pepper to taste.

Instructions:
1. Lay the entire wheat tortilla or wrap level on a perfect surface.
2. Spread the hummus equitably over the tortilla, leaving a little line around the edges.
3. Layer the store turkey bosom cuts, blended greens, destroyed carrots, and cut avocado (if using) on top of the hummus.
4. Season with salt and pepper to taste.

5. Crease in the sides of the tortilla and roll it up firmly into a wrap.

6. Slice the wrap down the middle askew, whenever wanted, and secure with toothpicks to maintain a reasonable level of control.

7. Serve right away or enclose it with material paper for a helpful in a hurry lunch choice.

8. Partake in your scrumptious and fulfilling turkey and hummus wrap!

Day2: Supper - Veggie Sautéed food with Tofu:

Ingredients:

- 1 block extra-firm tofu, squeezed and cubed -

2 tablespoons soy sauce or tamari - 1 tablespoon sesame oil

- 1 tablespoon olive oil

- 2 cloves garlic, minced

- 1 tablespoon ground ginger

- 2 cups blended vegetables, (for example, ringer peppers, broccoli, carrots, and snap peas), cut
- Cooked earthy colored rice or quinoa for serving - Sesame seeds and cut green onions for decorate.

Instructions:
1. In a bowl, throw the cubed tofu with soy sauce or tamari to equally cover.
2. Heat olive oil in an enormous skillet or wok over medium intensity. Add the marinated tofu 3D squares and cook until brilliant brown and firm on all sides. Eliminate from the skillet and put away.
3. In a similar skillet, add sesame oil and intensity over medium intensity. Add minced garlic and ground ginger, and sauté for 1-2 minutes until fragrant.
4. Add the cut blended vegetables to the skillet and sauteed for 5-7 minutes until delicate fresh.
5. Return the cooked tofu to the skillet and throw to join with the vegetables.

6. Serve the veggie pan sear with tofu over cooked earthy colored rice or quinoa.

7. Embellish with sesame seeds and cut green onions whenever wanted.

8. Partake in your delightful and nutritious veggie pan sear with tofu! Rehash the feast arranging and recipes for the leftover days of the week, changing piece sizes and fixings depending on the situation to meet your wholesome necessities and inclinations. Pay attention to your body, remain hydrated, and partake in a reasonable and differed diet to help your irregular fasting routine and wellbeing and prosperity.

Day 3: Breakfast - Banana Nut For the time being Oats:

Ingredients:
- 1/2 cup moved oats
- 1/2 cup unsweetened almond milk (or any milk of your decision)
- 1/2 ready banana, pounded
- 1 tablespoon chia seeds

- 1 tablespoon slashed nuts (like almonds, pecans, or walnuts)
- 1/2 teaspoon vanilla concentrate
- 1/2 teaspoon cinnamon
- Discretionary garnishes: cut banana, extra hacked nuts, sprinkle of honey or maple syrup.

Instructions:

1. In a Bricklayer container or water/air proof compartment, join moved oats, almond milk, squashed banana, chia seeds, cleaved nuts, vanilla concentrate, and cinnamon.

2. Mix well to join all fixings.

3. Cover the container or compartment and refrigerate for the time being, or for something like 4 hours, to permit the oats to mellow and the flavors to merge.

4. Toward the beginning of the day, give the short-term oats a mix and change the consistency with extra almond milk whenever wanted.

5. Serve the banana nut for the time, being oats cool, directly from the fridge, or

intensity them up in the microwave for a warm breakfast choice.

6. Top with cut banana, extra slashed nuts, and a sprinkle of honey or maple syrup, whenever wanted, prior to serving.

7. Partake in your delectable and helpful breakfast!

Day3: Lunch - Chickpea Salad Wraps:

Ingredients:
- 1 can (15 ounces) chickpeas, depleted and washed
- 1/4 cup plain Greek yogurt
- 1 tablespoon lemon juice
- 1 tablespoon cleaved new dill (or 1 teaspoon dried dill)
- 1/4 cup diced cucumber
- 1/4 cup diced red ringer pepper
- 1/4 cup diced red onion
- Salt and pepper to taste
- 2 entire wheat tortillas or wraps
- Leafy greens or spinach leaves for wrapping.

Instructions:

1. In a blending bowl, crush the chickpeas with a fork or potato masher until marginally thick.

2. Add Greek yogurt, lemon juice, hacked dill, diced cucumber, diced red ringer pepper, and diced red onion to the crushed chickpeas. Mix until very much merged.

3. Season the chickpea salad combination with salt and pepper to taste, changing flavoring depending on the situation.

4. Spread out the entire wheat tortillas or wraps on a perfect surface. Place a small bunch of leafy greens or spinach leaves in the focal point of every tortilla.

5. Spoon the chickpea salad and blend onto the greens, isolating it equally between the two tortillas.

6. Overlap in the sides of the tortillas and roll them up firmly into wraps.

7. Slice each wrap down the middle askew, whenever wanted, and secure with toothpicks to keep them intact.

8. Serve the chickpea salad wraps right away or envelop them with material paper for a convenient lunch choice. 9. Partake in your delightful and fulfilling chickpea salad wraps!

Day 3: Supper - Barbecued Chicken with Broiled Yams and Asparagus:

Ingredients:
- 2 boneless, skinless chicken bosoms - 2 tablespoons olive oil
- 2 cloves garlic, minced
- 1 teaspoon dried thyme
- Salt and pepper to taste
- 2 medium yams, stripped and cubed
- 1 pack asparagus, intense closures managed
- 1 tablespoon balsamic vinegar (discretionary)
- New parsley for embellish.

Instructions:

1. Preheat the barbecue to medium-high intensity.

2. In a little bowl, consolidate olive oil, minced garlic, dried thyme, salt, and pepper to make a marinade for the chicken.

3. Place the chicken bosoms in a shallow dish and pour the marinade over them, going to uniformly cover. Let marinate for somewhere around 15-30 minutes.

4. While the chicken is marinating, preheat the broiler to 400°F (200°C). Orchestrate the cubed yams on a baking sheet fixed with material paper.

5. Sprinkle the yams with olive oil and season with salt and pepper. Throw to cover uniformly, then, at that point, spread them out in a solitary layer.

6. Place the baking sheet in the preheated broiler and meal the yams for 20-25 minutes, or until delicate and gently caramelized, flipping partially through.

7. While the yams are broiling, barbecue the marinated chicken bosoms for 6-8 minutes

for each side, or until cooked through and presently not pink in the middle.

8. As of now of barbecuing, add the managed asparagus lances to the barbecue and cook until delicate, fresh and softly roasted.

9. Eliminate the chicken and asparagus from the barbecue and let rest for a couple of moments prior to cutting the chicken into strips.

10. Serve the barbecued chicken with cooked yams and barbecued asparagus.

11. Shower with balsamic vinegar, whenever wanted, and embellish with new parsley.

12. Partake in your nutritious and delightful supper! Rehash the dinner arranging and recipes for the leftover days of the week, changing part sizes and fixings depending on the situation to meet your nourishing requirements and inclinations. Pay attention to your body, remain hydrated, and partake in a reasonable and changed diet to help your discontinuous fasting routine and wellbeing and prosperity.

Day 4: Breakfast - Spinach and Mushroom Omelet:

Ingredients:
- 2 eggs
- 1/4 cup slashed spinach
- 1/4 cup cut mushrooms
- 1 tablespoon diced onion
- 1 tablespoon diced ringer pepper
- 1 tablespoon destroyed cheddar (like cheddar or feta)
- Salt and pepper to taste
- Cooking splash or olive oil for lubing the container.

Instructions:
1. In a little bowl, whisk the eggs until very much beaten. Season with salt and pepper to taste.
2. Heat a non-stick skillet over medium intensity and softly oil with cooking splash or olive oil.

3. Add the diced onion and ringer pepper to the skillet and sat for 2-3 minutes until mellowed.

4. Add the cut mushrooms to the skillet and cook for an extra 2-3 minutes until delicate.

5. Spread the cooked vegetables equitably across the lower part of the skillet.

6. Pour the beaten eggs over the vegetables, shifting the skillet to spread them out equitably.

7. Cook the omelet for 2-3 minutes, lifting the edges with a spatula and shifting the skillet to permit the uncooked egg to stream under.

8. When the base is set and the top is still somewhat runny, sprinkle the hacked spinach and destroyed cheddar equally north of one portion of the omelet.

9. Crease the other portion of the omelet over the filling to frame a half-moon shape.

10. Cook for another 1-2 minutes until the cheddar is softened, and the omelet is cooked through.

11. Cautiously slide the omelet onto a plate and serve hot.

12. Partake in your nutritious and tasty spinach and mushroom omelet!

Day 4: Lunch - Quinoa and Dark Bean Salad:

Ingredients:
- 1 cup cooked quinoa
- 1/2 cup canned dark beans, depleted and washed
- 1/2 cup diced tomatoes
- 1/4 cup diced red onion
- 1/4 cup hacked cilantro
- Juice of 1 lime
- 1 tablespoon olive oil
- Salt and pepper to taste
- Discretionary fixings: cut avocado, disintegrated feta cheddar, or tortilla strips.

Instructions:
1. In an enormous blending bowl, consolidate the cooked quinoa, dark beans,

diced tomatoes, diced red onion, and slashed cilantro.

2. In a little bowl, whisk together the lime juice, olive oil, salt, and pepper to make the dressing.

3. Pour the dressing over the quinoa and dark bean blend, throwing until all around merged.

4. Change preparing to taste, adding more salt, pepper, or lime juice whenever wanted.

5. Partition the quinoa and dark bean salad into individual serving bowls.

6. Embellish with discretionary fixings, for example, cut avocado, disintegrated feta cheddar, or tortilla strips, whenever wanted.

7. Serve chilled or at room temperature and partake in your reviving and fulfilling salad!

Day 4: Supper - Mediterranean Chicken Sticks with Tzatziki Sauce:

Ingredients: For the chicken sticks:
- 2 boneless, skinless chicken bosoms, cut into pieces

- 1 tablespoon olive oil
- 1 teaspoon dried oregano
- 1 teaspoon paprika
- 1/2 teaspoon garlic powder
- Salt and pepper to taste
- Cherry tomatoes, chime pepper pieces, and red onion lumps for spearing
- Wooden or metal sticks For the tzatziki sauce:
- 1/2 cup Greek yogurt
- 1/2 cucumber, ground and pressed to eliminate overabundance dampness
- 1 clove garlic, minced
- 1 tablespoon lemon juice
- 1 tablespoon cleaved new dill (or 1 teaspoon dried dill)
- Salt and pepper to taste.

Instructions:
1. With utilizing wooden sticks, absorb them water for no less than 30 minutes to forestall consuming.
2. In a bowl, join olive oil, dried oregano, paprika, garlic powder, salt, and pepper to make a marinade for the chicken.

3. String the marinated chicken pieces onto the sticks, substituting with cherry tomatoes, ringer pepper lumps, and red onion lumps.

4. Preheat a barbecue or barbecue container with medium-high intensity. Barbecue the chicken sticks for 4-5 minutes for each side, or until the chicken is cooked through and gently roasted.

5. While the chicken sticks are barbecuing, set up the tzatziki sauce. In a little bowl, consolidate Greek yogurt, ground cucumber, minced garlic, lemon juice, cleaved dill, salt, and pepper. Mix until all around merged.

6. Serve the barbecued chicken sticks with tzatziki sauce as an afterthought for plunging.

7. Partake in your delightful and fulfilling Mediterranean-propelled supper! Rehash the dinner arranging and recipes for the leftover days of the week, changing piece sizes and fixings on a case-by-case basis to meet your healthful requirements and inclinations. Pay attention to your body, remain hydrated, and partake in a decent and fluctuated diet to

help your irregular fasting routine and wellbeing and prosperity.

Day 5: Breakfast - Berry Protein Smoothie:

Ingredients:
- 1/2 cup frozen blended berries (like strawberries, blueberries, and raspberries)
- 1/2 banana, cut
- 1/2 cup unsweetened almond milk (or any milk of your decision)
- 1/2 cup plain Greek yogurt
- 1 scoop vanilla protein powder
- 1 tablespoon almond spread (or any nut margarine of your decision)
- Discretionary: honey or maple syrup to taste for added pleasantness.

Instructions:
1. Place the frozen blended berries, cut banana, almond milk, Greek yogurt, protein powder, and almond margarine in a blender.

2. Mix until smooth and rich, adding more almond milk if necessary to arrive at your ideal consistency.

3. Taste the smoothie and add honey or maple syrup on the off chance that you favor a better flavor, mixing again to integrate.

4. Empty the berry protein smoothie into a glass and appreciate right away.

5. Alternatively, decorate with extra berries or a sprinkle of granola for added surface.

6. Partake in your reviving and protein-stuffed breakfast smoothie!

Day5: Lunch - Chickpea and Veggie Buddha Bowl:

Ingredients: For the chickpeas:
- 1 can (15 ounces) chickpeas, depleted and flushed
- 1 tablespoon olive oil
- 1 teaspoon smoked paprika
- 1/2 teaspoon garlic powder
- Salt and pepper to taste

For the buddha bowl:
- Cooked quinoa or earthy colored rice
- Leafy greens or spinach leaves
- Cut cucumber
- Cherry tomatoes, divided
- Cut avocado
- Hummus for sprinkling
- Lemon wedges for crushing

Instructions:
1. Preheat the stove to 400°F (200°C). Line a baking sheet with material paper.
2. In a blending bowl, through the depleted and washed chickpeas with olive oil, smoked paprika, garlic powder, salt, and pepper until uniformly covered.
3. Spread the carefully prepared chickpeas out on the pre-arranged baking sheet in a solitary layer.
4. Cook the chickpeas in the preheated stove for 20-25 minutes, mixing part of the way through, until firm and brilliant brown.

5. While the chickpeas are cooking, set up the excess elements for the buddha bowl.

6. To gather the buddha bowl, begin with a base of cooked quinoa or earthy colored rice in a serving bowl.

7. Organize blended greens or spinach leaves, cut cucumber, divided cherry tomatoes, cut avocado, and cooked chickpeas on top of the quinoa or rice.

8. Shower with hummus and press lemon wedges over the bowl for added character.

9. Serve the chickpea and veggie buddha bowl right away and partake in your nutritious and fulfilling lunch!

Day 5: Supper - Turkey Taco Lettuce Wraps:

Ingredients:
- 1 tablespoon olive oil
- 1 pound ground turkey
- 1 parcel taco preparing blend
- 1/2 cup water

- Chunk of ice lettuce leaves, washed and dried
- Garnishes: diced tomatoes, diced avocado, destroyed cheddar, cleaved cilantro, Greek yogurt or acrid cream, salsa.

Instructions:

1. Heat olive oil in a skillet over medium intensity. Add ground turkey and cook until sauteed, splitting it up with a spatula as it cooks.

2. When the turkey is cooked through, add taco preparing blend and water into the skillet. Mix to merge.

3. Stew the turkey combination for 5-7 minutes, or until the sauce thickens and covers the meat.

4. Eliminate the skillet from intensity and let the turkey combination cool marginally.

5. To gather the lettuce wraps, spoon a part of the turkey combination onto every lettuce leaf.

6. Top with diced tomatoes, diced avocado, destroyed cheddar, hacked cilantro, Greek yogurt or acrid cream, and salsa as wanted.

7. Serve the turkey taco lettuce wraps right away, with additional garnishes as an afterthought.

8. Partake in your tasty and low-carb supper choice! Rehash the dinner arranging and recipes for the leftover days of the week, changing piece sizes and fixings depending on the situation to meet your dietary necessities and inclinations. Pay attention to your body, remain hydrated, and partake in a decent and shifted diet to help your irregular fasting routine and wellbeing and prosperity.

Day 6: Breakfast - Veggie Omelet:

Ingredients:
- 2 eggs
- 2 tablespoons diced ringer pepper
- 2 tablespoons diced onion
- 2 tablespoons diced tomato
- 2 tablespoons hacked spinach
- 1 tablespoon destroyed cheddar (discretionary)

- Salt and pepper to taste
- Cooking splash or olive oil for lubing the dish.

Instructions:

1. In a little bowl, beat the eggs until very much merged. Season with salt and pepper to taste.

2. Heat a non-stick skillet over medium intensity and daintily oil with cooking shower or olive oil.

3. Add the diced chime pepper and onion to the skillet and sauté for 2-3 minutes until mellowed.

4. Add the diced tomato and cleaved spinach to the skillet and cook for an extra 1-2 minutes until the spinach withers.

5. Spread the cooked vegetables equally across the lower part of the skillet.

6. Pour the beaten eggs over the vegetables, shifting the skillet to spread them out uniformly.

7. Cook the omelet for 2-3 minutes, lifting the edges with a spatula and shifting the

skillet to permit the uncooked egg to stream under.

8. When the base is set and the top is still marginally runny, sprinkle the destroyed cheddar equitably north of one portion of the omelet (if using).

9. Crease the other portion of the omelet over the filling to frame a half-moon shape.

10. Cook for another 1-2 minutes until the cheddar is dissolved, and the omelet is cooked through.

11. Cautiously slide the omelet onto a plate and serve hot.

12. Partake in your nutritious and delightful veggie omelet!

Day 6: Lunch - Quinoa and Dark Bean Stuffed Ringer Peppers:

Ingredients:
- 2 enormous chime peppers, divided and seeds eliminated
- 1 cup cooked quinoa

- 1 cup canned dark beans, depleted and washed
- 1/2 cup diced tomatoes
- 1/4 cup diced red onion
- 1/4 cup slashed cilantro - Juice of 1 lime
- 1 teaspoon ground cumin
- Salt and pepper to taste
- Destroyed cheddar for fixing (discretionary)

Instructions:

1. Preheat the broiler to 375°F (190°C). Place the split chime peppers in a baking dish.

2. In an enormous blending bowl, consolidate the cooked quinoa, dark beans, diced tomatoes, diced red onion, cleaved cilantro, lime juice, ground cumin, salt, and pepper. Mix until very much merged.

3. Spoon the quinoa and dark bean combination uniformly into each chime pepper half, pushing down delicately to pack the filling.

4. With utilizing destroyed cheddar, sprinkle it over the stuffed ringer peppers.

5. Cover the baking dish with aluminum foil and heat in the preheated stove for 25-30 minutes, or until the chime peppers are delicate.

6. Eliminate the foil and heat for 5 extra minutes to soften the cheddar (if using) and daintily brown the tops.

7. Eliminate from the broiler and let cool somewhat prior to serving.

8. Serve the quinoa and dark bean stuffed ringer peppers hot, decorated with extra slashed cilantro whenever wanted.

9. Partake in your healthy and fulfilling lunch!

Day 6: Supper - Heated Cod with Lemon Garlic Spread Sauce:

Ingredients: - 2 cod filets
- 2 tablespoons unsalted spread, liquefied
- 2 cloves garlic, minced
- Zing of 1 lemon - Juice of 1/2 lemon

- 1 tablespoon slashed new parsley
- Salt and pepper to taste

Instructions:

1. Preheat the stove to 375°F (190°C). Line a baking sheet with material paper.

2. Put the cod filets on the pre-arranged baking sheet.

3. In a little bowl, join softened spread, minced garlic, lemon zing, lemon juice, cleaved parsley, salt, and pepper.

4. Spoon the lemon garlic to spread sauce over the cod filets, covering them uniformly.

5. Heat in the preheated broiler for 12-15 minutes, or until the cod is dark and pieces effectively with a fork.

6. Eliminate from the stove and let cool somewhat prior to serving.

7. Serve the heated cod with extra lemon wedges as an afterthought for pressing.

8. Partake in your tasty and nutritious supper! Rehash the feast arranging and recipes for the leftover days of the week, changing part sizes and fixings depending on the situation to meet your nourishing

requirements and inclinations. Pay attention to your body, remain hydrated, and partake in a reasonable and fluctuated diet to help your discontinuous fasting routine and wellbeing and prosperity.

Day 7: Breakfast - Peanut Butter Banana Smoothie:

Ingredients:
- 1 ready banana
- 1 tablespoon peanut butter
- 1/2 cup unsweetened almond milk (or any milk of your decision)
- 1/4 cup plain Greek yogurt
- 1 tablespoon honey or maple syrup (discretionary)
- Small bunch of ice blocks

Instructions:
1. Strip the ready banana and break it into pieces.
2. In a blender, join the banana lumps, peanut butter, almond milk, Greek yogurt,

honey or maple syrup (if using), and ice solid shapes.

3. Mix until smooth and rich, changing the consistency with more almond milk if necessary.

4. Taste the smoothie and add more honey or maple syrup for added pleasantness whenever wanted.

5. Pour the peanut butter banana smoothie into a glass and appreciate right away.

6. Alternatively, embellish with a shower of peanut butter or a sprinkle of crushed peanuts for additional character.

7. Partake in your heavenly and stimulating breakfast smoothie!

Day 7: Lunch - Mediterranean Chickpea Salad:

Ingredients:
- 1 can (15 ounces) chickpeas, depleted and washed
- 1/2 cucumber, diced

- 1/2 cup cherry tomatoes, split - 1/4 cup diced red onion - 1/4 cup slashed new parsley
- 2 tablespoons additional virgin olive oil
- 1 tablespoon lemon juice
- 1 teaspoon dried oregano
- Salt and pepper to taste
- Disintegrated feta cheddar for garnish (discretionary)

Instructions:

1. In an enormous blending bowl, join the chickpeas, diced cucumber, cherry tomatoes, diced red onion, and slashed parsley.

2. In a little bowl, whisk together the additional virgin olive oil, lemon juice, dried oregano, salt, and pepper to make the dressing.

3. Pour the dressing over the chickpea salad and prepare until very much joined.

4. Change preparing to taste, adding more salt, pepper, or lemon juice whenever wanted.

5. Move the chickpea salad to individual serving bowls or plates. 6. Top with disintegrated feta cheddar, if using, for added character.

7. Serve the Mediterranean chickpea salad chilled or at room temperature.

8. Partake in your reviving and supplement stuffed lunch!

Day 7: Supper - Barbecued Vegetable Quinoa Bowls:

Ingredients:
- 1 cup cooked quinoa
- Grouped vegetables for barbecuing, (for example, zucchini, ringer peppers, eggplant, and cherry tomatoes)
- 2 tablespoons olive oil
- Salt and pepper to taste
- Lemon wedges for serving
- Discretionary garnishes: disintegrated feta cheddar, slashed new spices, balsamic coating

Instructions:

1. Preheat the barbecue to medium-high intensity.

2. Cut the varying vegetables into uniform pieces for barbecuing.

3. In a huge blending bowl, throw the cut vegetables with olive oil, salt, and pepper until very much covered.

4. Organize the carefully prepared vegetables on the preheated barbecue and cook for 5-7 minutes on every side, or until delicate and gently singed.

5. While the vegetables are barbecuing, heat the cooked quinoa if necessary and split it between serving bowls.

6. When the vegetables are barbecued however you would prefer, eliminate them from the barbecue and let cool somewhat.

7. Organize the barbecued vegetables on top of the quinoa in each bowl.

8. Press lemon wedges over the dishes for added newness.

9. Decorate with discretionary fixings, for example, disintegrated feta cheddar, cleaved

new spices, or a sprinkle of balsamic coating, whenever wanted.

10. Serve the barbecued vegetable quinoa bowls right away.

11. Partake in your delightful and bright supper! Rehash the dinner arranging and recipes for the leftover days of the week, changing piece sizes and fixings on a case-by-case basis to meet your dietary necessities and inclinations. Pay attention to your body, remain hydrated, and partake in a reasonable and shifted diet to help your irregular fasting routine and wellbeing and prosperity.

- Stress The executives and Rest Cleanliness.

Stress the executives and rest cleanliness are fundamental parts of keeping up with prosperity and supporting a solid way of life, particularly while consolidating irregular fasting. Here are a few systems for successfully overseeing pressure and advancing better rest:

1. Care and Unwinding Strategies:

- Practice care reflection, profound breathing activities, or moderate muscle unwinding to lessen feelings of anxiety and advance unwinding.

- Integrate exercises, for example, yoga or judo into your daily schedule, which can assist with quieting the psyche and further develop rest quality.

2. Customary Activity:

- take part in customary actual work, like energetic strolling, running, or strength preparing, to lessen pressure and further develop rest.

- Hold back nothing 30 minutes of moderate activity most days of the week, however keep away from enthusiastic exercises near sleep time, as they might obstruct rest.

3. Smart dieting Propensities:

- Keep a reasonable eating routine wealthy in natural products, vegetables, entire grains, and lean proteins to help wellbeing and prosperity.

- Keep away from exorbitant caffeine, liquor, and weighty or zesty dinners, particularly at night, as they can disturb rest designs.

4. Laying out a Loosening up Sleep time Schedule:

- Make a predictable sleep time routine to show to your body that now is the ideal time to slow down and plan for rest.

- Take part in quieting exercises before bed, like perusing, cleaning up, or paying attention to relieving music.

5. Restricting Screen Time:
- Lessen openness to electronic gadgets, for example, cell phones, tablets, and PCs, basically an hour prior to sleep time, as the blue light transmitted can obstruct the body's normal rest wake cycle.
- Consider using blue light channels or night mode settings on gadgets to limit openness to invigorating light.

6. Establishing an Agreeable Rest Climate:
- Keep your room cool, calm, and dim to advance better rest. Consider using power outage shades, earplugs, or a background noise if essential.
- Put resources into an agreeable bedding and pads that help your resting position and inclinations.

7. Overseeing Pressure and Tension:

- Distinguish wellsprings of stress in your life and foster procedures to adapt to them successfully, for example, critical thinking, looking for social help, or rehearsing positive self-talk.
- Consider merging unwinding strategies or care rehearses over the course of the day to oversee pressure and advance a feeling of quiet.

8. Looking for Proficient help if necessary:
- On the off chance that pressure or rest hardships continue regardless of self improvement techniques, consider looking for help from a psychological well-being proficient, for example, a specialist or instructor, who can give customized direction and backing. By integrating these pressure the executives methods and rest cleanliness rehearses into your day to day daily schedule, you can uphold your general wellbeing and prosperity while exploring the difficulties of discontinuous fasting. Recollect that consistency and persistence are critical, and rolling out slow

improvements after some time can prompt enduring enhancements in feelings of anxiety and rest quality.

Chapter Eight
Future Headings in Irregular Fasting Exploration.

Future bearings in discontinuous fasting research are probably going to investigate a few vital regions to additionally figure out its consequences for wellbeing and prosperity. A few expected areas of the center might include:

1. Long haul Wellbeing Results: Proceeded with research is expected to examine the drawn out impacts of discontinuous fasting on different wellbeing results, including metabolic wellbeing, cardiovascular wellbeing, mental capability, and life span. Enormous scope longitudinal examinations and randomized controlled preliminaries can give important bits of knowledge into the supported advantages and expected dangers of discontinuous fasting overstretched periods.

2. Ideal Fasting Conventions: Further exploration is expected to decide the best and practical discontinuous fasting conventions for various populaces and ailments. This remembers investigating varieties for fasting span, recurrence, and timing, as well as customized approaches in view of individual factors like age, sex, hereditary qualities, and way of life.

3. Components of Activity: More profound comprehension of the fundamental natural systems through which irregular fasting applies its belongings can give important experiences to its possible restorative targets. Exploration might zero in on explaining atomic pathways engaged with metabolic guideline, cell fix processes, safe capability, and chemical flagging pathways impacted by fasting.

4. Influence on Unambiguous Ailments: Examining the job of discontinuous fasting in the anticipation and the executives of explicit medical issue, like weight, type 2 diabetes, cardiovascular illness, neurodegenerative problems, and disease, is

fundamental. Clinical preliminaries focusing on these populaces can assist with deciding the viability and wellbeing of discontinuous fasting mediations.

5. Mix Treatments: Investigating the synergistic impacts of joining irregular fasting with other way of life mediations, like activity, dietary alterations, and pharmacotherapy, may offer novel methodologies for advancing wellbeing results and sickness anticipation. Exploration might zero in on recognizing reciprocal techniques that upgrade the advantages of discontinuous fasting while limiting expected unfavorable impacts.

6. Viability in Various Populaces: Examining the adequacy of discontinuous fasting across assorted populaces, including people of various ages, identities, financial foundations, and wellbeing situations with, urgent for guaranteeing its materialness and openness to a wide scope of people.

7. Conduct and Psychosocial Variables: Understanding the social and psychosocial factors that impact adherence to

discontinuous fasting regimens can educate the improvement regarding viable techniques to help conduct change and advance long haul adherence. Exploration might investigate factors like inspiration, self-guideline, social help, and social effects on fasting conduct.

8. Moral and Cultural Ramifications: Thought of the moral, social, and cultural ramifications of advancing irregular fasting as a way of life mediation is fundamental. Examination might investigate issues connected with value, admittance to medical care assets, social acknowledgment, and likely potentially negative side-effects of broad reception of fasting rehearses. By tending to these examination needs, researchers can propel how we might interpret discontinuous fasting and its job in advancing wellbeing and prosperity, eventually illuminating clinical practice rules and general wellbeing proposals later on.

- Arising Studies and Areas of Interest.

Arising studies and areas of interest in discontinuous fasting research are constantly developing as researchers investigate new roads and extend how we might interpret its impacts on wellbeing and prosperity. Probably the most recent Time-Confined Eating (TRE): Late examination has zeroed in on time-confined eating, a type of irregular fasting that limits everyday food admission to a particular window of time (e.g., 8-10 hours) trailed by a fasting period. Studies have explored the impacts of various eating windows on metabolic wellbeing, weight on the board, and circadian rhythms. 2. Fasting-Imitating Diets (FMDs): Fasting-emulating abstains from food include devouring low-calorie, plant-based dinners intended to impersonate the physiological impacts of fasting while as yet giving fundamental supplements. Arising studies have analyzed the likely advantages of

FMDs for life span, cell recovery, and infection anticipation.

3. Discontinuous Fasting and Stomach Microbiota: Exploration has shown that irregular fasting might significantly affect the piece and variety of the stomach microbiota, which assumes a basic part in processing, safe capability, and wellbeing. Arising studies are investigating the systems hidden by these impacts and their suggestions for metabolic wellbeing and sickness.

4. Discontinuous Fasting and Maturing: Studies have recommended that irregular fasting might apply hostile to maturing impacts by advancing cell fix, decreasing irritation, and improving pressure opposition pathways. Arising research intends to additionally explain the sub-atomic components included and investigate the capability of irregular fasting as a life span advancing intercession.

5. Discontinuous Fasting and Mind Wellbeing: Developing proof recommends that irregular fasting might make

neuroprotective impacts and upgrade mental capability by advancing brain adaptability, decreasing oxidative pressure, and balancing neuroinflammation. Arising studies are examining the capability of irregular fasting to forestall age-related mental deterioration and neurodegenerative illnesses like Alzheimer's and Parkinson's.

6. Irregular Fasting and Disease: Starter research proposes that discontinuous fasting might have anticancer impacts by restraining cancer development, upgrading chemotherapy viability, and lessening malignant growth risk factors like aggravation and insulin obstruction. Arising studies are investigating the capability of discontinuous fasting as an adjunctive treatment for disease counteraction and treatment.

7. Irregular Fasting in Clinical Populaces: Scientists are progressively concentrating on the impacts of discontinuous fasting in unambiguous clinical populaces, incorporating people with corpulence, type 2 diabetes, cardiovascular sickness, and

immune system problems. Arising concentrates on plan to explain the wellbeing, viability, and likely components of irregular fasting mediations in these populaces.

8. Discontinuous Fasting and Psychological wellness: There is developing interest in the impacts of irregular fasting on emotional wellness and close to home prosperity. Arising research recommends that irregular fasting might adjust synapse frameworks, further develop temperament guideline, and diminish side effects of wretchedness and nervousness. Further investigations are expected to investigate these impacts and their clinical ramifications. By tending to these arising areas of interest, researchers can extend how we might interpret discontinuous fasting and its likely applications for further developing wellbeing and prosperity across assorted populaces. Continuous exploration endeavors will keep on revealing insight into the systems fundamental the impacts of irregular fasting and illuminate the

improvement regarding proof based proposals for its utilization.

- Expected Applications in Safeguard Medication.

Discontinuous fasting holds guarantee as a potential preventive medication method because of its different physiological consequences for metabolic wellbeing, cell capability, and illness risk factors. A few likely utilizations of irregular fasting in preventive medication include:

1. Weight The executives: Irregular fasting can advance weight reduction by lessening calorie admission and working on metabolic productivity. It might likewise assist with forestalling weight recapture by improving fat digestion and protecting fit bulk, making it a significant device for overseeing corpulence and forestalling related unexpected problems like sort 2 diabetes, cardiovascular sickness, and certain tumors.

2. Metabolic Wellbeing: Discontinuous fasting has been displayed to work on different markers of metabolic wellbeing,

including insulin awareness, blood glucose levels, lipid profiles, and pulse. These impacts can help forestall or oversee metabolic problems like insulin opposition, prediabetes, metabolic condition, and non-alcoholic greasy liver sickness.

3. Cardiovascular Wellbeing: Irregular fasting might apply helpful consequences for cardiovascular wellbeing by decreasing irritation, oxidative pressure, and hazard factors for coronary illness, for example, hypertension, dyslipidemia, and stomach heftiness. It might likewise work on vascular capability, upgrade endothelial wellbeing, and lessen the gamble of atherosclerosis, myocardial localized necrosis, and stroke.

4. Type 2 Diabetes Avoidance: Irregular fasting has been displayed to further develop insulin awareness, lower fasting blood glucose levels, and lessen the gamble of creating type 2 diabetes. It might likewise assist with forestalling difficulties related to diabetes, like diabetic neuropathy, nephropathy, and retinopathy, by advancing

glycemic control and diminishing fundamental irritation.

5. Disease Counteraction: Primer proof recommends that discontinuous fasting might have likely anticancer impacts by hindering growth development, upgrading invulnerable reconnaissance, and sharpening malignant growth cells to chemotherapy and radiation treatment. It might likewise lessen malignant growth risk factors like heftiness, insulin opposition, persistent irritation, and oxidative pressure.

6. Neuroprotection: Discontinuous fasting has been displayed to advance mind wellbeing and brain adaptability by animating the development of neurotrophic factors, diminishing oxidative pressure, and improving mitochondrial capability. These impacts might assist with forestalling age-related mental deterioration, neurodegenerative sicknesses like Alzheimer's and Parkinson's, and state of mind problems like despondency and uneasiness.

7. Life span Advancement: Arising research proposes that discontinuous fasting might broaden life expectancy and improve health span by actuating cell stress reaction pathways, upgrading autophagy and DNA fix instruments, and decreasing age-related degenerative cycles. It might likewise defer the beginning old enough related illnesses and advance sound maturing by enhancing metabolic, hormonal, and fiery pathways.

8. Insusceptible Capability: Irregular fasting has been displayed to adjust resistant capability by advancing safe cell recovery, decreasing irritation, and improving invulnerable reconnaissance against microbes and malignant growth cells. It might assist with forestalling irresistible illnesses, immune system problems, and persistent fiery circumstances by advancing invulnerable reactions and keeping up with resistant homeostasis. By integrating irregular fasting into preventive medication methodologies, medical services suppliers can enable people to make proactive strides towards upgrading their wellbeing and

diminishing their gamble of creating constant infections. Further examination is expected to completely clarify the components fundamental the preventive impacts of irregular fasting and to foster proof based rules for its utilisation.

- Consolidating Customized Approaches.

Integrating customized ways to deal with discontinuous fasting can enhance its viability and security by fitting proposals to individual attributes, inclinations, and objectives. Here are a few different ways customized approaches can be coordinated:

1. Evaluation of Individual Wellbeing Status: Prior to beginning irregular fasting, people ought to go through an exhaustive appraisal of their wellbeing status, including clinical history, momentum prescriptions, metabolic profile, and hazard factors for constant illnesses. This evaluation can assist with recognizing any contraindications or extraordinary contemplations that might impact the decision of a fasting routine.

2. ID of Ideal Fasting Convention: Customized approaches include choosing the most reasonable fasting convention in view of individual factors, for example, age, sex, body structure, metabolic rate, action

level, and dietary propensities. A few people might blossom with more limited fasting windows (e.g., 16/8 strategy), while others might favor longer fasting periods (e.g., substitute day fasting) or more adaptable methodologies (e.g., time-confined eating).

3. Thought of Way of life and Timetable: Customized approaches consider an individual way of life variables and everyday schedules while planning fasting regimens. For instance, people with requesting work timetables or sporadic shift examples might profit from adaptable fasting plans that oblige their way of life requirements. Competitors and truly dynamic people might expect acclimations to their fasting conventions to upgrade execution and recuperation.

4. Checking and Criticism: Normal observing of progress and input from medical care suppliers or confirmed fasting mentors can assist people with changing their fasting regimens by considering their developing requirements and objectives. Objective measures, for example, body

weight, body synthesis, blood glucose levels, lipid profiles, and markers of metabolic wellbeing can give significant experiences into the adequacy of irregular fasting intercessions.

5. Wholesome Direction: Customized approaches incorporate individualized dietary direction to guarantee that people meet their supplement needs and keep up with satisfactory energy levels during fasting periods. This might include upgrading dinner timing, synthesis, and segment sizes to help metabolic wellbeing, muscle safeguarding, and prosperity. Enrolled dietitians or nutritionists can give customized dietary proposals considering individual inclinations and dietary examples.

6. Social Help: Integrating conduct support techniques, for example, objective setting, self-observing, responsibility, and critical thinking abilities can upgrade adherence to discontinuous fasting regimens and work with long haul conduct change. Social mediations custom fitted to individual necessities and inclinations can assist with

defeating boundaries to consistence and advance reasonable way of life alterations.

7. Incorporation with Other Restorative Modalities: Customized approaches might include coordinating discontinuous fasting with other helpful modalities like activity, stress the executives, rest cleanliness, and pharmacotherapy to improve wellbeing results and address explicit wellbeing concerns. Cooperative consideration groups can organize multidisciplinary intercessions customized to individual necessities and inclinations. By integrating customized approaches into irregular fasting mediations, medical services suppliers can engage people to arrive at informed conclusions about their wellbeing and prosperity, augment the advantages of fasting, and limit possible dangers. Fitting proposals to individual attributes and inclinations can upgrade adherence, fulfillment, and long haul accomplishment with discontinuous fasting regimens.

Conclusion

Enabling Yourself Through Information. Engaging yourself through information is fundamental while thinking about discontinuous fasting as a way of life mediation for wellbeing and prosperity. By grasping the standards, advantages, and potential dangers related to discontinuous fasting, you can pursue informed choices that line up with your singular objectives, inclinations, and wellbeing status. Throughout this investigation, we've dug into the science behind discontinuous fasting, looking at its impacts on digestion, weight for the executives, metabolic wellbeing, mental capability, and that's just the beginning. We've talked about different fasting conventions, reasonable tips for progress, and methodologies for conquering normal worries and confusions. We've additionally investigated raising research regions and customized ways to deal with irregular fasting, featuring the significance of fitting proposals to individual requirements, inclinations, and objectives. By coordinating customized approaches with proof based rehearses, you can upgrade the adequacy and wellbeing of irregular fasting while advancing long haul adherence and workable way of life changes. As you set out on your irregular fasting venture, recall that information is power. Remain inquisitive, remain informed, and remain associated with medical care experts or guaranteed fasting mentors who can give direction, support, and customized suggestions en route. Eventually, by enabling yourself through information and making proactive strides towards working on your wellbeing and prosperity, you can bridle the capability of discontinuous fasting to upgrade your personal satisfaction and accomplish your health objectives. Here's to an excursion of self-revelation, personal development, and self-strengthening through irregular fasting and then some.

- Synopsis of Key Focus points.

1. Figuring out Discontinuous Fasting: Irregular fasting includes rotating times of eating and fasting, with different conventions accessible to suit individual inclinations and objectives.

2. Advantages of Irregular Fasting: Discontinuous fasting can prompt weight reduction, worked on metabolic wellbeing, upgraded mental capability, and potential life span benefits.

3. Commonsense Tips for Progress: Begin steadily, remain hydrated, focus on supplement thick food varieties, pay attention to your body, and look for help from medical services experts or ensured fasting mentors.

4. Customized Approaches: Designer discontinuous fasting conventions to individual necessities, inclinations, and objectives, considering factors like a way of life, wellbeing status, and timetable.

5. Long haul Achievement: Spotlight on consistency, tolerance, and workable way of

life changes as opposed to handy solutions or momentary outcomes. 6. Assets for Additional Investigation: Use legitimate wellsprings of data, like logical diaries, books, online networks, and affirmed experts, to extend how you might interpret discontinuous fasting and backing your excursion towards better wellbeing and prosperity.

- Support for Long haul Achievement.

Embrace discontinuous fasting as a practical direction for living that lines up with your singular necessities and objectives. Remain committed, remain positive, and commend your advancement en route.

Recollect that each little step towards better wellbeing matters, and you can roll out enduring improvements for a better and more joyful life.

- Assets for Additional Investigation.

- Logical diaries and examination articles on discontinuous fasting and related points.

- Books by legitimate writers and specialists in sustenance, digestion, and irregular fasting.

- Online people group and gatherings where you can associate with other people who are investigating irregular fasting and offer encounters, tips, and backing.

- Confirmed medical care experts or fasting mentors who can give customized direction, backing, and proposals custom-made to your singular requirements and objectives. By utilizing these assets and remaining informed, you can keep on growing your insight, refine your way to deal with discontinuous fasting, and make long haul progress in your excursion towards better wellbeing and prosperity.